Nuclear Cardiology
Principles and Methods

Topics in Cardiovascular Disease

Series Editors:

Edmund Sonnenblick
Albert Einstein School of Medicine, New York

and

William W. Parmley
University of California Medical School, San Francisco

NUCLEAR CARDIOLOGY: Principles and Methods
Edited by Aldo N. Serafini, Albert J. Gilson, and William M. Smoak • 1976

Nuclear Cardiology
Principles and Methods

Edited by Aldo N. Serafini,
Albert J. Gilson, and William M. Smoak

*Mount Sinai Medical Center
and University of Miami School of Medicine
Miami, Florida*

Plenum Medical Book Company
New York and London

Library of Congress Cataloging in Publication Data

Main entry under title:

Nuclear cardiology.

(Topics in cardiovascular disease)
Includes bibliographical references and index.
1. Cardiovascular system–Diseases–Diagnosis. 2. Radioisotopes in cardiology. 3.
Radioisotope scanning. I. Serafini, Aldo N. II. Gilson, Albert J. III. Smoak, William M.
IV. Series [DNLM: 1. Radioisotopes–Diagnostic use. 2. Heart diseases–Diagnosis.
3. Heart diseases–Physiopathology. WG 141 C641]
WG141 C641]

RC669.C53	616.1'07'575	76-39783
ISBN 0-306-30952-1		

© 1977 Plenum Publishing Corporation
227 West 17th Street, New York, N. Y. 10011

Plenum Medical Book Company is an imprint of Plenum Publishing Corporation

Printed in the United States of America

Contributors

Naomi P. Alazraki, Departments of Radiology and Medicine, University of California, Medical Center, San Diego, California

David R. Allen, Department of Cardiology and Nuclear Medicine, Veterans Administration Hospital, Seattle, Washington

William L. Ashburn, Division of Nuclear Medicine, Department of Radiology, University of California Medical Center, San Diego, California

Fuad S. Ashkar, Department of Radiology, University of Miami School of Medicine, Jackson Memorial Hospital, Miami, Florida

Frederick J. Bonte, Department of Radiology, Southwestern Medical School, The University of Texas Health Science Center, Dallas, Texas

Gary Brock, Departments of Radiology and Medicine, University of California Medical Center, San Diego, California

L. Maximilian Buja, Department of Pathology, Southwestern Medical School, The University of Texas Health Science Center, Dallas, Texas

George C. Curry, Department of Radiology, Southwestern Medical School, The University of Texas Health Science Center, Dallas, Texas

James H. Ellis, Jr., Department of Medicine, Denver Veterans Administration Hospital, University of Colorado Medical Center, Denver, Colorado

Milton T. English, Department of Cardiology and Nuclear Medicine, Veterans Administration Hospital, Seattle, Washington

Ronald D. Finn, Department of Radiology, Baumritter Institute of Nuclear Medicine, Mount Sinai Medical Center, Miami Beach, Florida

Albert J. Gilson, Department of Radiology, Baumritter Institute of Nuclear Medicine, Mount Sinai Medical Center, Miami Beach, Florida

K. Lance Gould, Department of Cardiology and Nuclear Medicine, Veterans Administration Hospital, Seattle, Washington

J. J. Greenberg, Department of Thoracic Surgery, University of Miami School of Medicine, Mount Sinai Medical Center, Miami Beach, Florida

Glen W. Hamilton, Nuclear Medicine and Cardiology Services and Department of Cardiology and Nuclear Medicine, Veterans Administration Hospital, Seattle, Washington

Hartmut Henning, Departments of Radiology and Medicine, University of California Medical Center, San Diego, California

Frank J. Hildner, Department of Medicine, University of Miami School of Medicine, Miami, Florida; and Department of Cardiology, Mount Sinai Medical Center, Miami Beach, Florida

J. E. Holden, Department of Radiology, University of Wisconsin Medical School, Madison, Wisconsin

Homer B. Hupf, Department of Radiology, Baumritter Institute of Nuclear Medicine, Mount Sinai Medical Center, Miami Beach, Florida

Warren R. Janowitz, Department of Radiology, Baumritter Institute of Nuclear Medicine, Mount Sinai Medical Center, Miami Beach, Florida

Michael Jenkins, Departments of Medicine and Surgery, Denver Veterans Administration Hospital, University of Colorado Medical Center, Denver, Colorado

Allen D. Johnson, Departments of Radiology and Medicine, University of California Medical Center, San Diego, California

J. Ward Kennedy, Nuclear Medicine and Cardiology Services and Veterans Administration Hospital, Seattle, Washington

P. J. Kenny, Department of Radiology, Baumritter Institute of Nuclear Medicine, Mount Sinai Medical Center, Miami Beach, Florida

Dennis Kirch, Departments of Medicine and Surgery, Denver Veterans Administration Hospital, University of Colorado Medical Center, Denver, Colorado

A. J. Kiuru, Department of Radiology, University of Wisconsin Medical School, Madison, Wisconsin

Gerry Maddoux, Departments of Medicine and Surgery, Denver Veterans Administration Hospital, University of Colorado Medical Center, Denver, Colorado

P. J. Nelson, Department of Radiology, University of Wisconsin Medical School, Madison, Wisconsin

R. J. Nickles, Department of Radiology, University of Wisconsin Medical School, Madison, Wisconsin

George Pappas, Departments of Medicine and Surgery, Denver Veterans Administration Hospital, University of Colorado Medical Center, Denver, Colorado

Robert W. Parkey, Department of Radiology, Southwestern Medical School, The University of Texas Health Science Center, Dallas, Texas

R. E. Polcyn, Department of Radiology, University of Wisconsin Medical School, Madison, Wisconsin

James L. Ritchie, Department of Cardiology and Nuclear Medicine, Veterans Administration Hospital, Seattle, Washington

R. R. Sankey, Department of Radiology, Baumritter Institute of Nuclear Medicine, Mount Sinai Medical Center, Miami Beach, Florida

Heinrich R. Schelbert, Departments of Radiology and Medicine, University of California Medical Center, San Diego, California

Aldo N. Serafini, Department of Radiology, Baumritter Institute of Nuclear Medicine, Mount Sinai Medical Center, Miami Beach, Florida

William M. Smoak, III, Department of Radiology, University of Miami School of Medicine, Baumritter Institute of Nuclear Medicine, Mount Sinai Medical Center, Miami Beach, Florida

Peter P. Steele, Department of Medicine, Denver Veterans Administration Hospital, University of Colorado Medical Center, Denver, Colorado

Ernest M. Stokely, Department of Radiology, Southwestern Medical School, University of Texas Health Science Center, Dallas, Texas

D. M. Tamer, Department of Pediatrics, University of Miami School of Medicine, Jackson Memorial Hospital, Miami, Florida

John W. Verba, Departments of Radiology and Medicine, University of California Medical Center, San Diego, California

Manuel Viamonte, Jr., Department of Radiology, University of Miami School of Medicine, and Mount Sinai Medical Center, Miami Beach, Florida

Maria Viamonte, Department of Pathology, University of Miami School of Medicine, and Mount Sinai Medical Center, Miami Beach, Florida

Denny D. Watson, Department of Radiology, Baumritter Institute of Nuclear Medicine, Mount Sinai Medical Center, Miami Beach, Florida

James T. Willerson, Department of Medicine, Southwestern Medical School, The University of Texas Health Science Center, Dallas, Texas

Barry L. Zaret, Departments of Internal Medicine and Diagnostic Radiology, Yale University School of Medicine, New Haven, Connecticut

Foreword

Nuclear medicine is undergoing major orientation both practically and conceptually. To this point nuclear medicine has directed the major portion of its effort to visualization of static organ systems. The true value of this technique lies not in its ability to graphically display organ systems, but rather its ability to measure organ function in a noninvasive manner.

Dr. Serafini and his colleagues have, in this book, brought together the experts of the different phases of cardiodynamics. The contents lead one to believe that there are relatively simple innocuous tests that can supply large amounts of extremely important physiologic data without the necessity for open invasion of the heart. Perhaps the most exciting part of the studies is the glimpse into the future they provide.

The depth and versatility of these techniques is displayed by the surprising variety of problems amenable to nuclear medicine examination.

Perhaps the one point that is ever present in all these techniques is the ability to perform the tests sequentially in different time frames as the patient's condition changes or a major event is taking place, such as surgery.

The work presented in this volume must be considered the genesis of the new nuclear medicine and I, for one, look forward with great anticipation to what will follow.

Albert J. Gilson

Preface

Recent advances in nuclear medicine have resulted in the development of a new field—nuclear cardiology. Because of new radiopharmaceuticals, new types of equipment, and improved techniques, a new dimension to the evaluation of the cardiac patient is being provided to the armamentarium of the practicing clinician. The rapid advances being made are a result of a multidisciplinary approach, with specialists from various fields contributing. This cooperation and teamwork is evident from the backgrounds of the various contributors in this book. The majority of the chapters in this volume describe nuclear cardiac techniques that can be safely and rapidly performed. As such, they have a great potential of providing a noninvasive method of evaluating the cardiac status of patients in whom cardiac disease is suspected. They will play an important complementary role to currently available diagnostic tests in the screening and staging of cardiac disease as well as provide an easily repeatable method of follow-up once therapy has been initiated, whether this is surgical or medical. It is hoped that this book will stimulate and promote further research and investigation in this dynamic new field and further improve our clinical techniques to the benefit of the cardiovascular patient.

Aldo Serafini

Contents

Part IV
Evaluation of Ventricular Function

Part V
Radioimmunoassay

Part I · Fundamentals

Basic Anatomy of the Normal and Diseased Heart

Manuel Viamonte, Jr. and Maria Viamonte

Conventional chest roentgenography, angiocardiography, and cast corrosion preparation studies of the heart have been supplemented by anatomical sections of cadavers in the horizontal, sagittal, and coronal planes. The heart is the most important anatomical structure of the middle mediastinum. The ventral coronal section of the heart (Figure 1) exhibits, from left to right, the superior vena cava (above), the right atrium (below) the ascending aorta (in the middle), the pulmonary trunk (to the right), and the right ventricle (below the aorta and pulmonary trunk). The dorsal coronal section of the heart (Figure 2) shows the bifurcation of the trachea (above) with the right and left primary divisions of the pulmonary trunk (in front of the main bronchi) and the pulmonary veins and left atrium (below). Above the right main bronchus one sees the arch of the azygos vein and above the left main bronchus, the arch of the aorta.

The right border of the heart on frontal chest roentgenograms is formed by the superior vena cava and the right atrium. In adults with a dilated and/or elongated thoracic aorta, the ascending aorta overlaps the superior vena cava and may project to the right of the cava (Figure 3). In infants, the right heart border may be partially or completely covered by the right lobe of the thymus gland.

The left heart border has three arches: (1) the aortic arch (a posterior structure slightly to the left of the thoracic spine); (2) the middle arch, which is formed primarily by the left border of the pulmonary trunk, by the left auricular appen-

MANUEL VIAMONTE, JR. · Department of Radiology and MARIA VIAMONTE · Department of Pathology, University of Miami School of Medicine, and Mount Sinai Medical Center, Miami Beach, Florida.

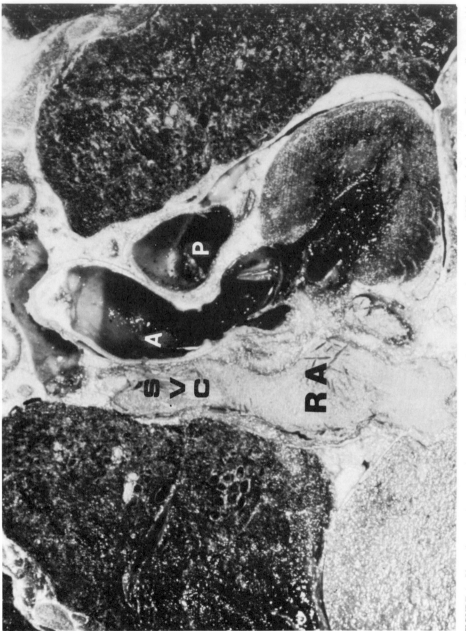

FIGURE 1. Ventral coronal section of the heart. Note from left to right: superior vena cava (SVC) and right atrium (RA); ascending aorta (A); and pulmonary trunk (below A and P).

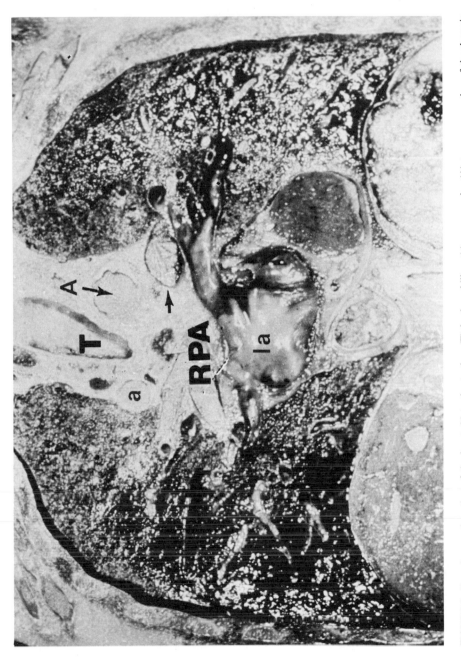

FIGURE 2. Dorsal coronal section of the heart. Note the trachea (T) in the midline; (a) azygos vein; (A) transverse portion of the thoracic aorta; the horizontal arrow indicates the left pulmonary artery; (RPA) right pulmonary artery; (la) left atrium.

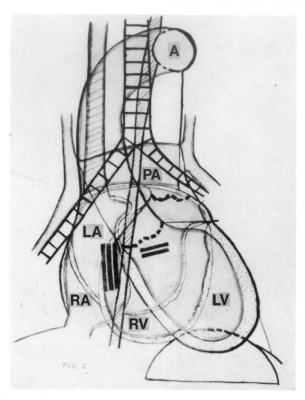

FIGURE 3. Diagram of the frontal projection of the cardiac chambers. A = aorta, LA = left atrium, RA = right atrium, RV = right ventricle, LV = left ventricle, and PA = pulmonary artery.

dage below it, and by the left branch of the pulmonary trunk; and (3) the free wall of the left ventricle. In infants, the left lobe of the thymus will cover the aortic arch and often the middle arch of the left border.

Pseudocardiomegaly may appear in pectus excavatum and in the so-called "straight-back syndrome." The heart may adopt the shape of a pancake. Lateral views of the chest and physical examination will distinguish true cardiac enlargement from pseudocardiomegaly caused by a thoracic deformity.

The second view of the heart, the left anterior oblique view (Figure 4), is taken at an angle of approximately 45° to the patient. In this view, the plane of the interatrial and interventricular septa appear almost in true profile. In front of the spine we find the left atrium and the left ventricle, and in front of these two chambers, the right atrium and the right ventrcle. *This is the view that separates the left from the right heart chambers.* It is the best view for assessing right atrial and left ventricular enlargements and septal defects.

The right anterior oblique view (Figure 5) is usually taken at 60°. In this obliquity, the posterior heart border usually clears the spine. Close to the spine are the left atrium (above), the right atrium (below), and the right ventricle and the left ventricle (in front). *This is the view that separates the atria from the ventricles* and is utilized for studying the atrioventricular valves. In the right anterior oblique view, usually obtained with a barium swallow, the atrioventricular valves can be seen in profile. This is the best view for assessing left atrial enlargement. The normal esophagus courses parallel to the thoracic spine; it may appear posteriorly displaced from left atrial enlargement. Enlargement of the right ventricle and occasionally the left ventricle may displace the left atrium dorsally. Therefore, disruption of the parallelism of the esophagus and the thoracic spine is indicative of left atriomegaly.

The left lateral view of the chest complements the information obtained from the right anterior oblique projection. In this view, the left side of the patient should be against the film or the plane of the image intensifier to provide minimum magnification of the cardiac silhouette. Posteriorly are the left atrium and the left ventricle and anteriorly, the right ventricle and the right atrium. The most anterior cardiac chamber is the right ventricle and the most posterior cardiac chamber is the left atrium. Demonstration of ventricular enlargement is impossible with minimal pressure-hypertrophy situations. Electrocardiography is more

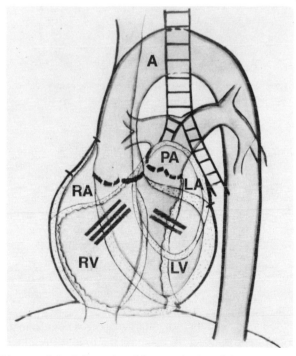

FIGURE 4. Diagram of the left anterior oblique projection of the cardiac chambers (45°). A = aorta, LA = left atrium, RA = right atrium, RV = right ventricle, LV = left ventricle, and PA = pulmonary artery.

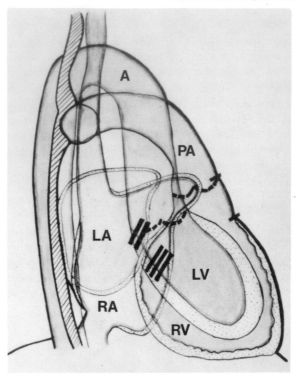

FIGURE 5. Diagram of the right anterior oblique projection of the cardiac chambers (60°). A = aorta, LA = left atrium, RA = right atrium, RV = right ventricle, LV = left ventricle, and PA = pulmonary artery.

sensitive than conventional roentgenography for the evaluation of early ventricular hypertrophies. When there is volume hypertrophy of any of the chambers, alteration of the cardiac contour will be observed.

Enlargement of the cardiovascular silhouette may be related to intrinsic dilatation of the heart, to pericardial effusion, or to juxtacardiac masses. Simpler than angiocardiography is the use of ultrasonography and radionuclide angiocardiography (Figure 6). Ultrasonography, complemented by radionuclide studies, will detect pericardial effusions. Scans with gallium-67 may be positive in pericardial effusion secondary to a malignant process involving the pericardium. The heart is surrounded by fat, and a prominent pleural pericardial fat pad may mimic cardiomegaly.

The best method to differentiate an enlarged azygos vein from a solid mass, such as an enlarged azygos node, is to compare frontal upright with frontal supine chest roentgenograms (Figure 7). In the former situation, the size of the density will increase in the supine position. Fluoroscopy will assist in this dif-

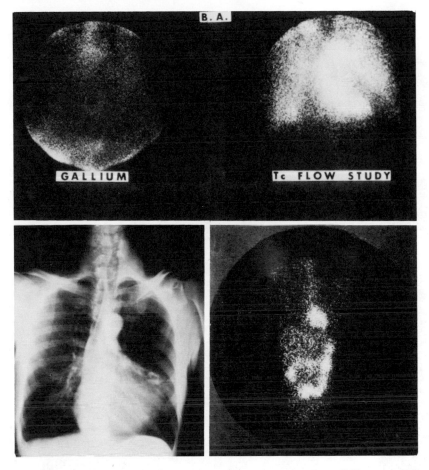

FIGURE 6. Use of radionuclides for assessing cardiac enlargement. Top—Gallium scan (left) and technetium flow study (right) on a patient with simple pericardial effusion. Note the radiolucent halo surrounding the heart, which is indicative of pericardial effusion. Bottom left—patient with bronchial carcinoma adjacent to the left cardiac border. Bottom right—Gallium study showing uptake at the level of the lung and the heart. Involvement of the pericardium by a bronchial carcinoma was confirmed.

ferential diagnosis, and is useful for the study of the thoracic aorta, ventricular contractility, and pulmonary hila. High-kilovoltage (120 kV or more) chest roentgenography offers the greatest anatomical information on the mediastinum. It will allow recognition of any displacement of the pleuro-azygo-esophageal line, which represents the medial extension of the right lower lobe in front of the thoracic spine (Figure 8). Left atriomegalies and retrocardiac masses will displace the pleuro-azygo-esophageal line laterally (Figure 9).

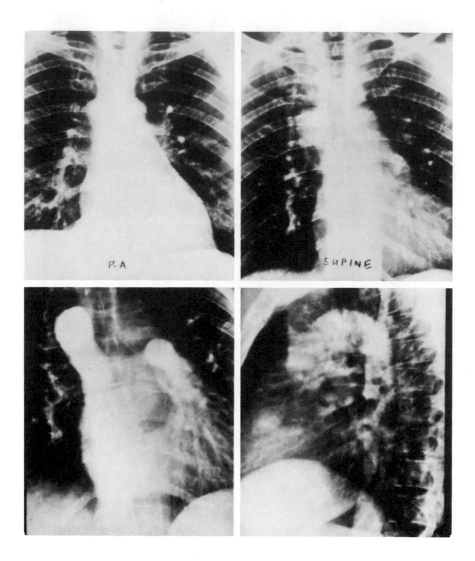

FIGURE 7. Azygos continuation of the inferior vena cava. Top left—frontal view of the chest showing a rounded density to the right of the trachea (vascular? mass?). Top right—same case; film obtained with the patient supine. Enlargement of the right paratracheal density supports the vascular nature of this process. Bottom left and right—Inferior vena cavogram showing opacification of a markedly enlarged azygos vein. The inferior vena cava is connected with the azygos system in the abdomen. There was agenesis of the hepatic segment of the inferior vena cava (azygos continuation of the inferior vena cava). The patient had no other anomalies.

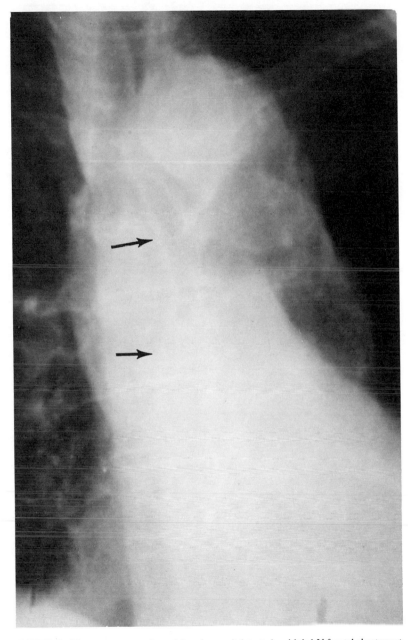

FIGURE 8. Pleuro-azygo-esophageal line (arrows) detected on high-kV frontal chest roentgenogram. Note how it descends vertically in front of the vertebral bodies. The right half of the vertebral bodies appear grayer than the left half due to the overlapping right lower lobe behind the heart and in front of the spine.

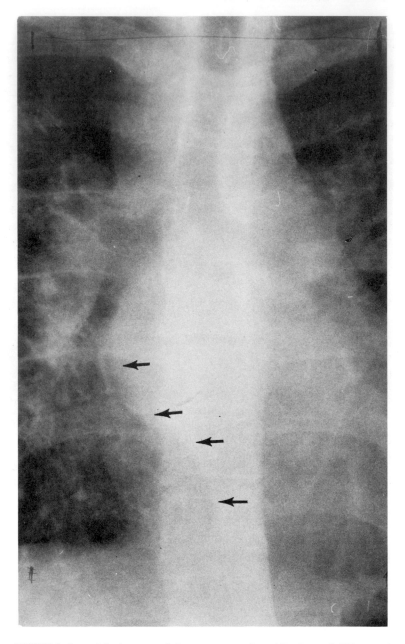

FIGURE 9. Lateral displacement of pleuro-azygo-esophageal line (arrows). This type of displacement is most commonly seen with enlargement of the left atrium. In this case it was related to a large infracarinal nodes in a patient with sarcoidosis.

Barium swallow is essential for studying vascular rings. The position of the aortic arch is best documented in infants by esophagography.

Studies of the *abdominal viscera* will complement the examination of the chest. Occasionally, herniation of intraabdominal organs into the chest may mimic cardiac enlargement or even mediastinal tumors. A liver scan will outline the position of the liver. Intravenous pyelography or renal scan will demonstrate the position of the kidney. Pulmonary hypoplasias are often associated with intrathoracic herniations of abdominal viscera or eventrations of the diaphragm. Conventional roentgenography of the chest and of the abdominal organs usually differentiate significant from nonclinically significant congenital thoracic anomalies. The atrial situs can be predicted from the anatomical positions of the liver and the stomach, and the ventricular situs, by the positions of the aorta and the pulmonary trunk.

Assessment of Left Ventricular Function: Current Methods and Clinical Significance

Glen W. Hamilton and J. Ward Kennedy

Introduction

Methods of evaluating and understanding the contractile performance of the heart have been actively pursued during much of the past century. Bowditch[1] demonstrated the all-or-none law of the heart in 1871. From 1895 to 1915, Frank,[2] Straub,[3] Wiggers,[4] and Starling[5] developed the basic concept that the mechanical energy of contraction (systole) was dependent upon the fiber length at end-diastole. Based on the model of muscle contraction proposed by A. V. Hill,[6] numerous investigators[7] have developed quantitative methods for assessing the contractile state of the myocardium. Additionally, the effects of afterload (the resistance or impedance) were appreciated and quantitated.[7] These three factors (resting fiber length, contractile state, and afterload) are the basic concepts underlying the overall performance of the heart.

Unfortunately, neither fiber length or contractile state is easily quantitated, and this is especially true in patients with disease processes that affect the ventricle in a segmental or regional fashion—the most common one being ischemic heart disease. The development of quantitative contrast angiocardiography by Dodge et al.[8] and Arvidsson[9] has, however, provided a very useful clinical method for assessing left ventricular pump function in humans. Ventricular volume measurements coupled with ventricular pressure provide an adequate method for assessing ventricular performance, which has become the one most

GLEN W. HAMILTON and J. WARD KENNEDY·Nuclear Medicine and Cardiology Services, Veterans Administration Hospital, Seattle, Washington.

commonly used. The systolic ejection fraction (SEF), in particular, has proved to be a valuable indicator of ventricular function in a wide variety of cardiac diseases. The recent development of noninvasive radionuclide methods for determining ventricular volumes and ejection fraction promises an even wider application of these methods. The angiographic methods currently used to obtain these data, how they vary with different cardiac diseases, and their predictive prognostic value in patients form the bases for the following discussion.

Quantitative Contrast Angiocardiography

Contrast left ventriculography is performed at the time of cardiac catheterization, often in conjunction with coronary angiography. Contrast material, 50–70 cc, is injected into the left ventricle through a catheter, and X-ray filming (single plane or biplane) is performed with a cine system or a rapid (12/sec) large film changer. Proper catheter selection, positioning, and timing of the onset of injection to end-diastole are used to minimize the occurrence of ventricular premature contractions. Simultaneous records of left ventricular pressure, ECG, and film timing are made to relate the ventricular volumes to the cardiac cycle. Next, the left ventricle is traced from the films, and the length, wall thickness, and area of each frame are determined. Based on the ellipsoidal model of Dodge et al.,[8] ventricular volume and left ventricular mass are determined in the manner described below.

The respective diameter D is determined from the planimetered area A and its maximal length L_m as follows:

$$D/2 = 2A/\pi L_m \tag{1}$$

The left ventricular volume V is then determined using the formula for the volume of an ellipsoid:

$$V = \tfrac{4}{3}\pi D_a/2 \times D_l/2 \times L_m/2$$

where D_a and D_l are the diameters determined from Eq. (1) for the anterior and lateral planes and L_m is the maximal length in either the lateral or anteroposterior plane. All measurements are corrected for X-ray magnification.

Calculated volumes are then corrected by a regression equation developed by X-ray studies of postmortem hearts distended with known volumes of contrast material:

$$V_{true} = V_{calc.} \ (0.928) - 3.8 \ \text{ml} \tag{3}$$

Left ventricular mass is determined by calculating the volume of the chamber plus the wall (V_{c+w}):

$$V_{c+w} = \tfrac{4}{3}\pi\left(\frac{D_a}{2} + T_u\right)\left(\frac{D_l}{2} + T_w\right)\left(\frac{L_m}{2} + T_w\right) \qquad (4)$$

where T_w is the measured thickness of the left ventricular wall. Then

$$\text{Left ventricular weight} = (V_{c+w} - V_{true})$$

$$\times \text{ muscle specific gravity (1.050)} \qquad (5)$$

From these data, a time–volume curve is constructed and end-diastolic volume (EDV) and end-systolic volumes (ESV) are determined.

Basic Calculations and Normal Values

The systolic ejection fraction represents the fraction of end-diastolic volume ejected during each beat by the ventricle, or the stroke volume (SV) divided by the end-diastolic volume:

$$SV = EDV - ESV \qquad (6)$$

$$EF = \frac{SV}{EDV} = \frac{EDV - ESV}{EDV} \qquad (7)$$

The total left ventricular output (CO) can be obtained by multiplying stroke volume by heart rate:

$$\text{Stroke volume (cc)} \times \text{heart rate (beats/min)} = CO \text{ (cc/min)} \qquad (8)$$

In patients with valvular regurgitation at the aortic or mitral valves, the difference between angiographic cardiac output and forward cardiac output determined by Fick or dye techniques represent the amount of regurgitation flow:

$$\frac{CO_{angio} - CO_{Fick}}{CO_{angio}} = \text{regurgitant flow fraction} \qquad (9)$$

Normal values for left ventricular volumes, ejection fraction, and left ventricular mass are shown in Table 1.

TABLE 1

Left ventricular end-diastolic volume	.70±20 ml/M^{2a}
Left ventricular end-systolic volume	.24±10 ml/M^2
Left ventricular stroke volume	.45±13 ml/M^2
Systolic ejection fraction	.0.67±0.08
Left ventricular mass	.76 g/M^2 (women) and 99 g/M^2 (men)
Left ventricular wall thickness	.8.9 mm (women) and 11.9 mm (men)

^{a}M^2 = meter squared body surface area.

Accuracy of the Angiocardiographic Method

With good-quality films, the reproducibility in calculating EDV by several observers is excellent. Barium-filled hearts measured by X ray and water displacement give essentially identical results. The calculation of ESV is often more difficult due to irregular ventricular contour and variations in the concentration of contrast material due to displacement by the papillary muscles and trabeculae. Nonetheless, stroke volume, calculated from (EDV − ESV = SV), correlates well with the stroke volume determined by other methods in the absence of valvular regurgitation.[10] Volumes calculated from single-plane anterior or right anterior oblique views correlate reasonably well with biplane volume calculations; $r = 0.88$ and 0.91, respectively.[11] Ventricular volumes and ejection fraction also vary in a single patient due to ventricular loading or unloading, catecholamine stimulation, heart rate and blood pressure changes, and other factors affecting contractility or afterload. It is thus critically important that measurements be made under reasonably stable and reproducible hemodynamic states.

Overall, it is our opinion that angiocardiographic ejection fraction measured at rest during cardiac catheterization is representative of true ventricular performance with reasonable limits; i.e., a measured EF is within ±15% of the true value, or an EF of 0.67 represents true ejection fraction of from 0.57 to 0.77. We thus consider an ejection fraction below 0.55 as probably abnormal, and an EF below 0.50 as certainly abnormal.

Parenthetically, I expect that noninvasive radionuclide methods are potentially more accurate than angiocardiographic methods when the radionuclide techniques are adequately developed. This may be particularly true in patients with segmental contraction abnormalities, in which the ventricle is often not ellipsoidal.

Alteration of Ventricular Volumes, Ejection Fraction, and Mass with Cardiac Disease

Changes in ventricular performance can be divided conveniently into several categories: (1) volume overload, (2) pressure overload, (3) myocardial disease, and (4) volume underload. Often there is a combination of abnormalities due to one or several disease processes. Table 2 summarizes these types of functional abnormalities and the usual causative or associated disease.

Generally, the changes in volume and mass can be considered as compensatory mechanisms to maintain stroke volume and, hence, cardiac output at normal or near-normal levels. Ejection fraction represents the ability or integrity of the ventricular contractile mechanisms and is a measure of the functional state of the cardiac muscle per se.

In patients with ventricular volume overload due to regurgitant valvular lesions, ventricular dilatation and hypertrophy occur to maintain forward SV at normal levels. Ventricular dilatation with EDVs of 3 (or more) times normal frequently occur. Left ventricular wall thickness increases only moderately (Figure 1), but mass increases greatly, due mainly to the large EDV. EF remains in the normal range until late in the course of the disease, and a reduced EF is cause to suspect additional myocardial disease.

Ventricular pressure overload causes little change in ventricular volumes or ejection fraction. The major change is myocardial hypertrophy with marked increases in left ventricular wall thickness and mass.

Myocardial disease is characterized by a primary decrease in contractile function, manifested as a decrease in ejection fraction. To compensate for the decreased EF, the ventricle dilates (usually accompanied by mild hypertrophy) and is often able to maintain SV at near-normal levels. Clinically, the onset of congestive heart failure usually coincides at an EF below 0.40.[12] It is helpful to note that in the absence of volume or pressure overload, cardiac enlargement (noted from physical examination or chest X ray) is always associated with a significantly reduced EF. Ventricular dysfunction with coronary disease represents a common and special form of myocardial disease characterized by regional dysfunction and will be discussed further.

Volume underload or impaired ventricular filling is seen primarily with mitral valve obstruction and constrictive pericarditis. Generally, volumes, EF, and mass are mildly reduced. The combination of diminished EF with normal or reduced EDV is extremely helpful in differentiating constrictive pericardial disease from primary myocardial disease.

Left ventricular function in coronary heart disease is characterized by re-

TABLE 2

Type of abnormality	Usual associated diseases
1. Volume overload	Mitral or aortic regurgitation, any cause
2. Pressure overload	Aortic stenosis, systemic hypertension
3. Myocardial disease	Atherosclerotic, myocardiopathy
4. Volume underload	Mitral stenosis, constrictive pericarditis

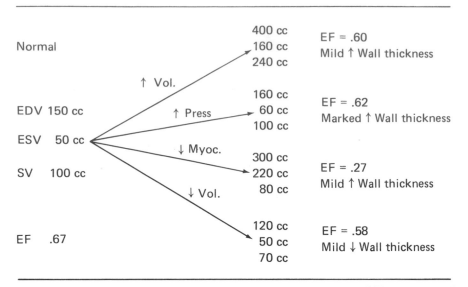

FIGURE 1. Typical changes in cardiac volumes and ejection fraction due to volume overload, pressure overload, myocardial disease, and volume underload.

gional contraction abnormalities. Contraction plots constructed by superimposition of the EDV and ESV drawings are useful in understanding this disease and can be graded as to type and severity,[12] as shown in Table 3.

The relationship of EF, contraction pattern, and left ventricular end-diastolic pressure is shown in Figure 2. Patients with chronic angina and no history of infarction usually have grade I or grade II contraction patterns, normal or minimally reduced EF, and no manifestations of heart failure. Conversely, patients with reduced EF and abnormal contraction patterns (III, IV, or V) have virtually all had previous infarction, and those with an EF below 0.40 usually have experienced congestive heart failure.[12] A summary of ventricular function in 67 patients with coronary disease is presented in Figure 3. Patients without previous infarction have normal ventricular contraction (EF) and ventricular filling (ED pressure and EDV). Most of the group with moderately diminished SEF but normal EDV have had infarction, but do not have congestive heart failure. The group of patients with markedly reduced EF have inordinate increases in EDV, and virtually all have had a previous infarction and congestive heart failure.

EF as a Predictive Factor in Coronary and Valvular Heart Disease

Studies published in the last two years have been helpful in clarifying the role of left ventricular dysfunction on survival in patients with ischemic heart

TABLE 3

Grade		Contraction abnormalities
I.	Normal	Normal symmetrical contraction
II.	Borderline	Borderline asymmetrical contraction involving less than 25% of ventricle
III.	Segmental abnormality	Akinetic or hypokinetic regions involving greater than 25% of ventricle
IV.	Segmental dyskinesis	Areas of ventricle with paradoxical motion
V.	Diffuse abnormality	Akinesis or hypokinesis involving greater than 75% of ventricle

disease. Data from 590 patients at the Cleveland Clinic, published by Bruschke *et al.*,[13] demonstrated that the presence of marked left-ventricular dysfunction in patients with single-vessel coronary disease was associated with a 60% 5-year mortality, compared to 7% in patients with normal left ventricular angiograms. In patients with three-vessel disease, a similar comparison revealed an increase in

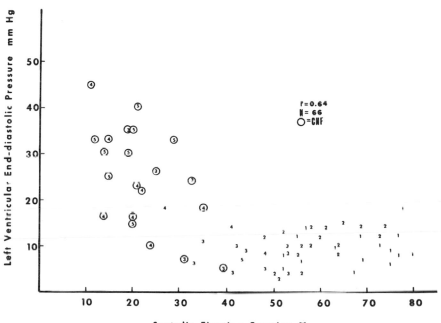

FIGURE 2. Relationship of systolic ejection fraction, left-ventricular end-diastolic pressure, and contraction pattern. The numbers refer to the contraction patterns outlined in Table 3. The circles represent patients with clinical congestive heart failure.

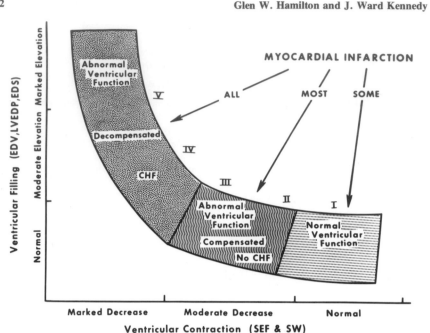

FIGURE 3. Overall relationship of contraction pattern, myocardial infarction, and parameters of ventricular filling and contraction: (SEF) systolic ejection fraction; (SW) stroke work; (EDV) end-diastolic volume; (LVEDP) left ventricular end-diastolic pressure; (EDS) end-diastolic stress.

5-year mortality from 36 to 88%. Murray et al.[14] in a recent report from this center, showed that medically treated patients with an ejection fraction of less than 40% had a 14-fold increase in mortality (28% per year) as compared to those with a normal ejection fraction (2% per year) over a 15-month follow-up period.

It is likely that there is a similar relationship between ejection fraction and prognosis in patients treated medically with valvular heart disease, although precise data are not currently available.

Several reports [15–18] are now available that relate left ventricular function as assessed by the ejection fraction to mortality during or soon after coronary artery bypass graft surgery. Operative mortality in the range of 1–4% is now expected in patients with normal ejection fraction (greater than 50%) and reasonable morphology of distal vessels, whereas perioperative mortality of over 30% can be expected in patients with an ejection fraction less than 30%, as shown in Table 4.

Effect of Cardiac Surgery on EF

A great deal of attention has been focused on the results of coronary bypass surgery on left ventricular function. Eight series comprising 352 patients with

TABLE 4. Effect of Left Ventricular Function on Operative Mortality
(Myocardial Revascularization)

Author	N	Ejection fraction	Operative mortality	
			High EF	Low EF
Oldham et al.[15]	87	0.25	4%	55%
Hammermeister and Kennedy[16]	138	0.33	3%	33%
Cohn et al.[17]	128	0.50	1%	29%
Yatteau et al.[18]	24	0.25		42%

stable angina pectoris are now available.[19-26] Only one of these studies showed an improvement in ejection fraction following surgery (53–63% in 46 patients). The mean ejection fraction in the entire group was 58% postoperatively. Of interest, in the series that demonstrated an increased ejection fraction, the patients were studied within 14 days following surgery, and heart rate and cardiac output were increased compared to their preoperative studies, suggesting that they had an elevated sympathetic response related to the stress of recent surgery.

Studies of left ventricular function before and following successful coronary artery bypass graft surgery in patients with unstable angina syndromes are limited at this time. Four reports,[21-23,27] totaling 28 patients, suggest that the ejection fraction may improve following surgery in these patients. The mean preoperative ejection fraction of 59% increased to 70% postoperatively. Unfortunately, follow-up studies in the majority of these patients were carried out in the early postoperative period.

At this time, it can be concluded from the experience reported from this and other institutions that successful coronary artery bypass grafting in patients with stable angina pectoris cannot be expected to improve left ventricular function as judged by the angiographic analysis of left ventricular ejection fraction. Approximately 20% of such patients may show some improvement, but an equal number will show a decrease in ejection fraction postoperatively. Patients studied during a period of unstable angina, especially if they have myocardial ischemia at the time of angiography, will more often demonstrate improved left ventricular performance on postoperative angiography, but such improvement cannot be expected in the majority.

We recently reported 1- to 3-year follow-up studies in patients with isolated aortic or mitral valve disease who had successful surgical treatment.[28] In 24 patients who had aortic valve replacement, end-diastolic volume, end-diastolic pressure, and left ventricular mass decreased significantly following surgery. In 15 patients with normal ejection fraction preoperatively, 14 remained normal at the postoperative evaluation. In the 9 patients with a low ejection fraction (less than 50%), 8 improved and 7 became normal postoperatively. These findings indicate that in patients with aortic valve disease, left ventricular function can be expected to improve or remain normal following valve replacement.

Similar evaluation of 19 patients with mitral valve disease has been reported.[29] In 12 patients with mitral stenosis (MS) or combined MS and mitral regurgitation (MR), despite excellent clinical results, there was no significant change in left ventricular end-diastolic pressure, volume, mass, or ejection fraction. In the 7 patients with MR alone, there was a significant increase in systolic pressure and a decrease in left ventricular end-diastolic pressure and volume. Left ventricular mass did not fall significantly, and the ejection fraction fell from $55 \pm 13\%$ to $43 \pm 16\%$. This experience indicates that valve replacement in patients with MR, although accompanied by a reduction in filling pressure and left ventricular volume, does not improve myocardial pump performance as judged by the ejection fraction.

Based on a change $\geq 10\%$ in the ejection fraction as the criterion for significant improvement or deterioration in left ventricular performance, the following conclusions can be drawn regarding the effects of surgery: In patients with ischemic heart disease, improvement in left ventricular function occurs in about 20%, is more likely in patients with unstable angina syndromes, and is balanced by a similar percentage of patients who developed significant deterioration in ejection fraction following surgery. In patients with valvular heart disease, those with aortic valve disease improve their ventricular pump function if it is abnormal preoperatively, those with MS show no improvement in left ventricular pump function, and those with isolated MR show a significant reduction in left ventricular ejection fraction following mitral valve replacement.

Summary

Quantitative angiocardiography has provided a useful method for assessing left ventricular function in humans. The systolic ejection fraction, in particular, is a valuable index of the contractile function of the cardiac muscle. Determination of ventricular volumes, mass, and ejection fraction provides a more comprehensive view of the hemodynamic alterations induced by various disease states. Additionally, the ejection fraction is a powerful indicator of prognosis during either medical or surgical therapy.

The major limitation of this method is the requirement for invasive cardiac catheterization with its attendant morbidity and occasional mortality. Second, the contrast angiocardiogram changes the hemodynamic state, making it difficult to use for assessing left ventricular function before and after various maneuvers (e.g., stress, nitroglycerin).

Radionuclide angiography overcomes the limitations and potentially offers data of equal or greater accuracy than contrast methods. The benefit to patients with cardiac disease is obvious, and radionuclide angiocardiography will very likely become one of the most common nuclear medicine procedures.

References

1. Bowditch, H. P., Ueber die Eigenthumlichkeiten der Reizbarkeit, welche die Muskelfasern des Herzens zeigen, *Verh. K. Sachs Ges. Wochenchnschr. Leipzig, Math. Physische,* C1 *23:*652 (1871).

2. Frank, O., Zur Dynamik des Herzmuskels, *Ztschr Bio. 32:*370 (1895) (trans. by C. B. Chapman and E. Wasserman), *Am. Heart J. 58:*282, 467 (1959).

3. Straub, H., Dynamik des Saugetierherzens: I. Dtsch. *Arch. Klin. Med. 115:*531 (1914); II. *116:*409 (1914).

4. Wiggers, C. J., Some factors controlling the shape of the pressure curve in the right ventricle, *Am. J. Physiol. 33:*382 (1914).

5. Starling, E. H., *The Linacre Lecture on the Law of the Heart,* Longmans, Green and Co., London (1918).

6. Hill, A. V., The heat of shortening and the dynamic constants of muscle, *Proc. R. Soc. London Ser.* B *126:*136 (1938).

7. Braunwald, E., *The Myocardium: Failure and Infarction,* H. P. Publishing Co., New York (1974).

8. Dodge, H. T., Sandler, H., Ballew, D. W., and Lord, Jr., J. D., The use of biplane angiocardiography for the measurement of left ventricular volume in man, *Am. Heart J. 60:*762 (1960).

9. Arvidsson, H., Angiographic determination of left ventricular volume, *Acta Radiol. 56:*321 (1961).

10. Hunt, D., Baxley, W. A., and Kennedy, J. W., *et al.,* Quantitative evaluation of cine aortography in the assessment of aortic regurgitation, *Am. J. Cardiol. 31:*696 (1973)

11. Kennedy, J. W., Trenholme, S. E., and Kasser, I. S., Left ventricular volume and mass from single-plane cineangiocardiogram. A comparison of anteroposterior and right anterior oblique methods, *Am. Heart J. 80:*343 (1970).

12. Hamilton, G. W., Murray, J. A., and Kennedy, J. W., Quantitative angiography in ischemic heart disease: The spectrum of abnormal left ventricular function and the role of abnormally contracting segments, *Circ. 45:*1065 (1972).

13. Bruschke, A. V. G., Proudfit, W. L., and Sones, F. M., Jr., Progress study of 590 consecutive nonsurgical cases of coronary disease followed by 5–9 years. II. Ventriculographic and other correlations, *Circ. 47:*1154 (1973).

14. Murray, J. A., Chinn, N., Peterson, D. R., Influence of left ventricular function on early prognosis in atherosclerotic heart disease, *Am. J. Cardiol. 33:* 159 (1974).

15. Oldham, H. N., Kong, Y., Bartel, A. G., Morris, J. J., Jr., Behar, V. S., Peter, R. H., Rosali, R. A., Young, G., Jr., and Sabiston, D. C., Risk factors in coronary artery bypass surgery, *Arch. Surg. 105:*918 (1972).

16. Hammermeister, K. E., and Kennedy, J. W., Predictors of surgical mortality in patients undergoing direct myocardial revascularization, *Circulation (Suppl. II) 50:*112 (1974).

17. Cohn, P. F., Gorlin, R., Cohn, L. H., and Collins, J. J., Jr., Left ventricular ejection fraction as a prognostic guide in surgical treatment of coronary and valvular heart disease, *Am. J. Cardiol. 34:*136 (1974).

18. Yatteau, R. F., Peter, R. H., Behar, V. S., Bartel, A. G., Rosali, R. A., and Kong, Y., Ischemic cardiomyopathy: The myopathy of coronary disease, *Am. J. Cardiol. 34:*520 (1974).

19. Rees, G., Bristow, J. D., Kremkau, E. L., Green, G. S., Herr, R. H., Griswold, H. E., and Stan, A., Influence of aortocoronary bypass surgery on left ventricular performance. *N. Engl. J. Med. 284:*1116 (1971).

20. Arbogast, R., Solignac, A., and Bourassa, M. G., Influence of aortocoronary saphenous vein bypass surgery on left ventricular volumes and ejection fraction, *Amer. J. Med. 54:*290 (1973).

21. Bolooki, H., Mallon, S., Ghahramani, A., Sommer, L., Vargas, A., Slavin, D., and Kaiser, G.

A., Objective assessment of the effects of aorto-coronary bypass operation on cardiac function, *J. Thorac. Cardiovasc. Surg. 66:*916 (1973).

22. Deal, P., Elliott, L. P., Bartley, T. D., Wheat, M. W., Jr, and Ramsey, H. W., Quantitative left ventriculography in the immediate postoperative period after aorto-coronary bypass, *J. Thorac. Cardiovasc. Surg. 66:*1 (1973).

23. Chatterjee, K., Swan, H. J. C., Parmley, W. W., Sustaita, H., Marcus, H. S., and Matloff, J., Influence of direct myocardial revascularization on left ventricular asynergy and function in patients with coronary heart disease, *Circulation 47:*276 (1973).

24. Hammermeister, K. E., Kennedy, J. W., Hamilton, G. W., Stewart, D. K., Gould, K. L., Lipscomb, K., and Murray, J. A., Aortocoronary saphenous vein bypass. Failure of successful grafting to improve resting left ventricular function in chronic angina, *N. Engl. J. Med. 290:*186 (1974).

25. Shepherd, R. L., Itscoitz, S. B., Glancy, D. L., Stinson, E. B., Reis, R. L., Olinger, G. N., Clark, C. E., and Epstein, S. E., Deterioration of myocardial function following aorto-coronary bypass operation, *Circ. 49:*467 (1974).

26. Seattle Heart Watch, unpublished data from J. A. Murray (1975).

27. Fischl, S. J., Herman, M. V., and Gorlin, R., The intermediate coronary syndrome. Clinical, angiographic and therapeutic aspects, *N. Engl. J. Med. 288:*1193 (1973).

28. Doces, J., Stewart, D., and Kennedy, J. W., Quantitative assessment of left ventricular function following successful aortic valve replacement, *Circulation* (Suppl. III to Vol. 49) *50:*21 (1974).

29. Doces, J., and Kennedy, J. W., Quantitative assessment of left ventricular function following successful mitral valve surgery, *Am. J. Cardiol. 35:*132 (1975).

Radiopharmaceuticals for Cardiovascular Investigations

Homer B. Hupf and Ronald D. Finn

The importance of imaging the myocardium lies in the possible benefit to the patient in the diagnosis and subsequent treatment of coronary artery disease. The rationale for the use of radionuclides in the evaluation of cardiovascular disease has not changed drastically over the past ten years. In the middle sixties, ^{86}Rb ($t_{1/2}$ = 18.66 days) was being investigated for myocardial infarct,[1] and ^{131}I ($t_{1/2}$ = 8.05 days) albumin was being evaluated for heart blood-flow studies.[2] Today, ^{81}Rb ($t_{1/2}$ = 4.7 hr) is being investigated for myocardial infarcts,[3-6] and ^{99m}Tc ($t_{1/2}$ = 6.05 hr) albumin is used for blood-flow studies.[7-8] The major improvements during the last decade have been the availability of more suitable radionuclides (many of which are cyclotron-produced), improved instrumentation (high-performance Anger cameras capable of isolating selected regions of interest), and the interfacing of computers with the cameras for data analyses. Myocardial scanning is not widely performed at the present time, since no completely satisfactory radiopharmaceutical has been available; however, extensive development work is currently underway, and the results to date are encouraging.

Computer-assisted heart blood-flow studies are used to locate aortic and ventricular aneurysms in single-pass studies or in ECG gated multiple-pass studies. Blood-flow studies with regions of interest and background subtraction are used to evaluate ejection fraction, shunts, and valvular insufficiencies. The main problem with the flow studies is obtaining statistically significant counts for proper interpretation, since a bolus will course through both sides of the heart in

HOMER B. HUPF and RONALD D. FINN · Department of Radiology, Baumritter Institute of Nuclear Medicine, Mount Sinai Medical Center, Miami Beach, Florida.

approximately 10 sec.[9] If ECG gating is utilized, the study is prolonged, since the camera is operative only for a portion of the time.

Myocardial perfusion studies are "static" images—if one can consider obtaining static images from a constantly moving organ. In these studies an absence of perfusion to an area of the myocardium in a resting individual usually indicates chronic or acute myocardial infarct, while a normal perfusion at rest and a defect after exercise indicate ischemia. The problems with this procedure include being able to identify a small defect in a dynamic organ and being able to differentiate between acute and chronic myocardial infarct, ischemia, and aneurysms. Currently, some positive imaging agents that tend to eliminate the problem of searching for a defect in a field of radioactivity are being evaluated for acute myocardial infarct. At the present time no one radiopharmaceutical can be utilized to answer all the questions, but, in general, one can list the properties a prospective agent should possess.

A high-concentration bolus is necessary to obtain a sufficient number of counts in a short time without a large diffusion of activity. Since the administered activity is usually high, a short-half-life nuclide is favored for a low dose to the patient. In addition, a short-half-life nuclide permits repeat studies when necessary. The nuclide should have a high photon abundance of an energy that is compatible with the imaging equipment. If the radiopharmaceutical is a chemical compound or a complex ion, it should remain intact and vascular during the course of the study. These latter properties are less important for single-pass flow studies.

The knowledge that certain monovalent cations accumulate in striated muscle and myocardium following intravenous injection has further spurred cardiovascular research. Included among these cations are potassium, which is the primary intracellular cation, and rubidium and cesium,[10] which are also members of Group I alkali metals. Other cations that have chemical behavior closely resembling these metals include the ammonium and thallium ions. Various complexes of technetium have also been reported as possibilities for identifying myocardial infarcts. Radioiodinated fatty acids are likewise reported to be potential intravenous myocardial imaging agents, since free fatty acids are major nutrients of the myocardium.

Potassium-43 has enjoyed the most development to date.[11-17] Normal myocardium contains exchangeable intracellular potassium, and the large dilution factor of the carrier-free radioactive potassium causes the radionuclide to remain in the myocardium sufficiently long for static imaging. Its disadvantages are its less than ideal decay characteristics for imaging and its currently high production cost.

Rubidium-82, obtained from a ^{82}Sr generator, is being evaluated.[18] Being a positron emitter, special instrumentation is necessary to obtain images with ^{82}Rb.[19]

The myocardial extraction of cesium as a potassium analogue has been studied with conflicting reports.[20-22] Some investigators claim a high and rapid extraction by the myocardium,[23] while others claim a low initial extraction.[24] At any rate, ^{129}Cs seems to offer little if any advantage over ^{43}K, and is equally expensive.

Reactor produced ^{134m}Cs, although contaminated with ^{134}Cs, has a good half-life for imaging, but short for distribution.[25] The photon energy is good for camera imaging, but of low abundance.

Several institutions with cyclotrons are evaluating ^{13}N-labeled ammonia, ammonium ion, and amino acids as myocardial imaging agents.[26-27] The incorporation of ammonia in the normal myocardium is thought to be a stepwise enzymatic amination of α-keto glutarate to glutamine.[28]The ammonium ion in ammonium chloride remains in the myocardium for approximately 1 hr, but accumulates in the liver and kidneys. The amino acid asparagine shows myocardial uptake several times higher than the alkali metals, while ^{13}N-labeled glutamine shows very little myocardial uptake.[29] Asparagine may therefore play a role in myocardial metabolism and be useful in the management of the cardiac patient. Special detection equipment designed for the 511-keV photon is necessary for imaging these compounds.

Thallium-201 appears to have an affinity for myocardial muscle and may be useful in identifying areas of ischemia and myocardial infarct.[30 32] In our limited experience it has demonstrated a good myocardial uptake with rapid blood clearance and little interference from surrounding tissues. It is cyclotron-produced and should be less expensive than ^{43}K. The high abundant 83-ke V X rays are adequate for camera imaging.

Several ^{99m}Tc complexes have been used for cardiovascular evaluations. Sodium pertechnetate appears to be a reasonable agent for single-pass computer-assisted flow studies. However, with the availability of a commercial kit for tagging albumin with ^{99m}Tc,* the albumin complex is superior, especially for multiple-pass studies, since it remains vascular for a longer period of time.

Polyphosphate, pyrophosphate, diphosphonate, tetracycline,[34] and glucoheptonate labeled with ^{99m}Tc are all being evaluated as positive imaging agents for acute myocardial infarcts. Several investigators[34,35] have compared these agents and found that all are concentrated to some degree in areas of acute myocardial infarct, but pyrophosphate and glucoheptonate show more rapid blood clearance, thus leading to a better myocardial infarct/normal myocardium ratio. Ratios between 35 and 7 have been reported for these agents.[35,36]

Unsaturated fatty acids, such as oleic acid, are metabolic agents for cardiac muscle, and the preparation of ^{99m}Tc-labeled oleic acid has been reported but not evaluated clinically.[37] ^{123}I-labeled fatty acids have been prepared and evaluated

*Supplied by New England Nuclear Corp., Boston, Massachusetts.

by Robinson et al.[38-40] Initial studies with ^{131}I-oleic acid[41-43] resulted in selective photoscans of the left ventricular muscle mass. Iodination of the double bond is apparently a metabolically recognizable change, and uptake is low. Increased uptakes are obtained when the double bond is left intact and the iodination occurs on a terminal carbon atom, such as in 16-iodo-9-hexadecenoic acid. We have evaluated this agent in our laboratory using normal and infarcted dogs. We find myocardial uptake complicated by accompanying lung uptake and fairly rapid metabolism. It is felt that the metabolism rate of fats by the myocardium is dependent on the degree of fasting and the level of blood sugar.[44] The disadvantages of ^{123}I compounds tend to be relatively high production costs and a lack of general availability.

Indium-113m, available from a [113]Sn generator, has also enjoyed some use.[45,46] Indium, when injected in the ionic form, apparently becomes bound to transferrin and can be used for flow studies. Indium bound to microspheres or macroaggregated albumin has also been injected directly into left and right coronary arteries to detect areas of constriction. Direct arterial injections are probably out of the scope of most nuclear medicine departments, but may be useful in conjunction with angiography or cardiac catheterization laboratories.

Table 1 lists some inorganic tracers currently being evaluated for myocardial infarcts and ischemia. With the exception of ^{67}Ga, all the nuclides in the table depict ischemia or infarct as filling defects with the inherent problems stated earlier.

Gallium-67 as the citrate, like the Tc-phosphates and tetracycline, is bound to acute myocardial infarcts, probably through the calcium deposited in the mitochondria.[34] It demonstrates a low myocardial infarct/normal myocardium

TABLE 1. Radioisotopes for Myocardial Imaging

Nuclide	Half-life	Photon energy in keV and abundance
[43]K	22.0 hr	373 (85%), 619 (81%), others
[81]Rb	4.7 hr	450, 511 (26%)
[82]Rb	1.3 min	511 (192%), 777 (9%)
[129]Cs	32.1 hr	375 (48%), 416 (25%)
[131]Cs	9.7 days	29 (88%)
[134m]Cs	2.9 hr	128 (14%)
[13]N	9.96 min	511 (200%)
[201]Tl	73.0 hr	69–83 (98%)
[99m]Tc	6.05 hr	140 (90%)
[123]I	13.3 hr	159 (83%)
[67]Ga	78.0 hr	93 (40%), 184 (24%), 296 (22%)
[113m]In	103 min	393 (64%)
[15]O	123 sec	511 (200%)

ratio, slow blood clearance, and high liver uptake[35]; however, it has the advantage of being readily available. Rubidium-81, another analogue of potassium, is undergoing extensive evaluation as the chloride for myocardial infarct.[10] An 80% extraction by the myocardium in one pass has been reported[47]; however, the disappearance from the myocardium is also rapid (V. J. Sodd, personal communication). The nuclide is cyclotron-produced, with a good half-life for heart studies, but poor for commercial distribution. As illustrated in Figure 1, it has the added feature of decaying to radioactive ^{81m}Kr, a diffusible tracer that offers the possibility of evaluating pulmonary function.

Most recently, the 2-min ^{15}O nuclide as labeled carbon dioxide is under extensive reevaluation at Mount Sinai Medical Center. When ^{15}O-labeled carbon dioxide is inhaled, it rapidly combines with water to form carbonic acid in the lung.[48] Carbonic anhydrase, present in the blood, hydrolyzes the carbonic acid, producing labeled water that dissolves in the blood, becoming a pulmonary vein injection. Production of O-15 at Mount Sinai Medical Center is accomplished by a recently developed pure oxygen gas target irradiated with protons. The oxygen labeled with ^{15}O is converted to carbon dioxide by a series of hot converters and delivered to the clinical area approximately 1 min after the end of bombardment.[49] The specific activity of the product is approximately 1.0 mCi/cc CO_2. The radiochemical purity is greater than 99.8%, as is the radionuclidic purity measured at end of bombardment. Figure 2 depicts the process schematically.

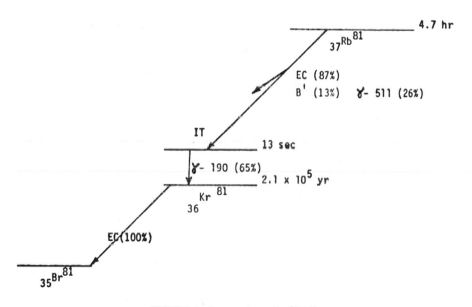

FIGURE 1. Decay scheme for ^{81}R.[50]

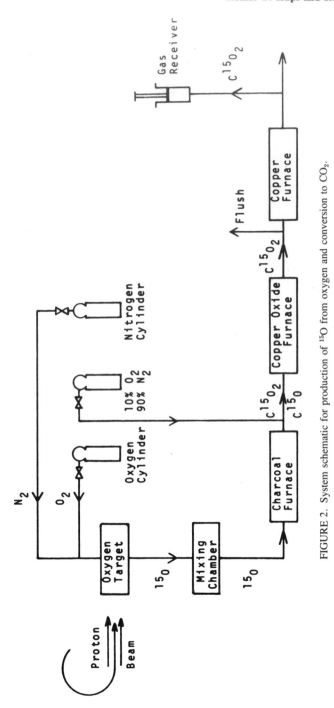

FIGURE 2. System schematic for production of ^{15}O from oxygen and conversion to CO_2.

Unquestionably, continued basic research and application of the knowledge gained by the use of existing radiopharmaceuticals will ultimately lead to improved patient care. The introduction and application of new radiopharmaceutic techniques to the evaluation of cardiovascular systems requires, however, that we initially understand the normal anatomical and physiological functions of the heart. Subsequent to this, we may then begin to apply our techniques to the diseased heart.

With the increasing sophistication of diagnostic tests, it behooves us as clinicians to understand not only the condition we are studying and evaluating, but also the means with which to choose to evaluate them.

In nuclear medicine, the availability of radiopharmaceuticals and photoscanning instrumentation is rapidly changing and adapting to our needs.

References

1. Carr, E. A., Jr., Beirwaltes, W. H. et al., Myocardial scanning with rubidium-86, J. Nucl. Med. 3:76 (1962).
2. Rejali, A. M., MacIntyre, W. J., et al., A radioisotope method for visualization of blood pools, Amer. J. Roentgenol. 79:129 (1958).
3. Budinger, T. F., McRae, J., et al., Myocardial imaging with Rb-81, J. Nucl. Med. 15:480 (1974) (abstract).
4. Harper, P. V., Rich, B., et al., Imaging studies with ^{81}Rb-^{81m}Kr (abstract), J. Nucl. Med. 15:500 (1974).
5. Lamb, J. F., Khentigan, A., et al., Rubidium-81 in evaluation of regional myocardial perfusion, (abstract) J. Nucl. Med. 15:509 (1974).
6. Martin, N. D., Zaret, B. L., et al., Rubidium-81, a new agent for myocardial perfusion scans at rest and exercise, and comparison with potassium-43 (abstract), J. Nucl. Med. 15:514 (1974).
7. Alpert, N. M., McKusick, K. A., et al., Noninvasive nuclear kinecardiography, J. Nucl. Med. 15:1182 (1974).
8. Watson, D. D., Sankey, R. R., et al., Cardiac Evaluation, Continuing Education Lectures, Southeastern Chapter, Society of Nuclear Medicine (November 1974).
9. Strauss, H. W., and Pitt, B., Cardiovascular nuclear medicine, Appl. Radiol. 4:57 (1975).
10. Watson, I. A., and Tilbury, R. S., Cyclotron production of the radionuclides ^{81}Rb, ^{82m}Rb and ^{129}Cs (abstract), J. Nucl. Med. 11:373 (1970).
11. Hurley, P. J., Cooper, M. C., et al., ^{43}KCl: A new radiopharmaceutical for imaging the heart, J. Nucl. Med. 12:516 (1971).
12. Skrabal, F., Glass, H. I., et al., A simplified method for simultaneous electrolyte studies in man utilizing potassium-43, Int. J. Appl. Radiat. Isot. 20:677 (1969).
13. Rhodes, B. A., Radiopharmaceuticals, in:Principles for Cardiovascular Nuclear Medicine (H. W. Strauss, et al., eds.) C. V. Mosley Co., St. Louis (1974).
16. Holman, B. L., Eldh, P., et al., Evaluation of myocardial perfusion after intracoronary injection of radiopotassium, J. Nucl. Med. 14:274 (1973).
17. Poe, N. D., Eber, L. M., et al., Evaluation of ^{43}K and ^{129}Cs for myocardial imaging (abstract), J. Nucl. Med. 14:440 (1973).
18. Grant, P. M., Erdal, B. R., et al., A ^{82}Sr-^{82}Rb isotope generator for use in nuclear medicine, J. Nucl. Med. 16:300 (1975).
19. Yano, Y., and Anger, H. P., Visualization of heart and kidneys in animals with ultrashort-lived ^{82}Rb and the positron scintillation camera, J. Nucl. Med. 9:412 (1968).

20. Carr, E. A., Gleason, G. *et al.*, The direct diagnosis of myocardial infarction by photoscanning after administration of cesium-131, *Amer. Heart J. 68:*627 (1964).

21. Yano, Y., VanDyke, D., *et al.*, Myocardial uptake studies with [129]Cs and the scintillation camera, *J. Nucl. Med. 11:*663 (1970).

22. Sodd, V. J., Blue, J. W. *et al.*, Cyclotron production of [129]Cs—a promising radiopharmaceutical, (abstract) *J. Nucl. Med. 11:*362 (1970).

23. Budinger, T. F., and Yano, Y., Myocardial function evaluated by uptake of Cs-129, (abstract) *J. Nucl. Med. 13:*417 (1972).

24. Poe, N. D., Comparative myocardial uptake and clearance characteristics of potassium and cesium, *J. Nucl. Med. 13:*57 (1972).

25. Chandra, R., Braunstein, P., *et al.*, [134m]Cs, A new myocardial imaging agent, *J. Nucl. Med. 14:*243 (1973).

26. Monaham, W. G., Tilbury, R. S. *et al.*, Uptake of ^{13}N-labeled ammonia, *J. Nucl. Med. 13:*274 (1972).

27. Harper, P. V., Lathrop, K. A., *et al.*, Clinical feasibility of myocardial imaging with [13]NH_3, *J. Nucl. Med. 13:*278 (1972).

28. Gelbard, A. S., Hara, T., *et al.*, Recent aspects of cyclotron production of medically useful radionuclides, in: *Radiopharmaceuticals and Labelled Compounds,* Vol. 1, IAEA, Vienna, 1973.

29. Gelbard, A. S., Clarke, L. P., *et al.*, Enzymatic synthesis and evaluation of N-13 labeled amino acids as myocardial scanning agents, (abstract) *J. Nucl. Med. 15:*492 (1974).

30. Kawana, M., Krizek, H. *et al.*, Use of [199]Tl as a potassium analog in scanning, (abstract) *J. Nucl. Med. 11:*333 (1970).

31. Lebowitz, E., Green, M. W. *et al.*, Thallium-201 for medical use, I., *J. Nucl. Med. 16:*151 (1975).

32. Bradley-Moore, P. R., Lebowitz, E. *et al.*, Thallium-201 for medical use, II: Biologic behavior, *J. Nucl. Med. 16:*156 (1975).

33. Holman, B. L., Dewanjee, M. K., *et al.*, Detection and localization of experimental myocardial infarction with ^{99m}Tc-tetracycline, *J. Nucl. Med. 14:*595 (1973).

34. Bonte, F. J., Parkey, R. W. *et al.*, Distribution of several agents useful in imaging myocardial infarcts, *J. Nucl. Med. 16:*132 (1975).

35. Zewiman, F. G., O'Keefe, A., *et al.*, Selective uptake of Tc-99m chelates and Ga-67 in acutely infarcted myocardium, (abstract) *J. Nucl. Med. 15:*546 (1974).

36. Rossman, D. J., Siegel, M. D., *et al.*, Accumulation of Tc-99m-glucoheptonate in acutely infarcted myocardium (abstract), *J. Nucl. Med. 15:*529 (1974).

37. Bonte, J. F., Graham, K. D. *et al.*, Preparation of Tc-99m-oleic acid complex for myocardial imaging (abstract), *J. Nucl. Med. 14:*381 (1973).

38. Poe, N. D., Robinson, G. D. *et al.*, Myocardial extraction of variously labeled fatty acids and carboxylates (abstract), *J. Nucl. Med. 14:*440 (1973).

39. Robinson, C. D., Jr., and Lee, A. W., Radioiodinated fatty acids for heart imaging: iodine monochloride addition compared with iodide replacement labeling, *J. Nucl. Med. 16:*17 (1975).

40. Poe, N. D., Robinson, G. D., *et al.*, Evaluation of 16 iodo-hexadeconoic acid as an indicator of regional myocardial perfusion (abstract), *J. Nucl. Med. 15:*524 (1974).

41. Evans, J. R., Gunton, R. W., *et al.*, Use of radioiodinated fatty acid for photoscans of the heart, *Circ. Res. 16:*1 (1965).

42. Gunton, R. W., Evans, J. R., *et al.*, Demonstration of myocardial infarction by photoscans of the heart in man, *Am. J. Cardiol. 16:*482 (1965).

43. Counsell, R. E., and Ice, R. D., *Design of Organ Imaging Radiopharmaceuticals,* p. 62, University of Michigan, Ann Arbor, (1973).

44. Schelber, H. R., Ashburn, W. L., *et al.*, Comparative myocardial uptake of intravenously administered radionuclides, *J. Nucl. Med. 15:*1092 (1974).

45. Berman, D. S., Salel, A. F. *et al.*, Non-invasive radioisotopic determination of cardiac output utilizing a single probe and a computer model (abstract), *J. Nucl. Med. 15:*478 (1974).
46. Hamilton, G. W., Ritchie, J. L. *et al.*, Detection of stress induced regional myocardial ischemia in humans by injection of MAA at rest and during contrast induced coronary hyperthermia (abstract), *J. Nucl. Med. 15:*499 (1974).
47. Peek, N. F., Hegedus, F. *et al.*, Rb-81 for myocardial studies (abstract), *J. Nucl. Med. 15:*522 (1974).
48. West, J. B., and Dollery, C. T., Uptake of oxygen-15 labeled CO_2 compared with carbon-11 labeled CO_2 in the lung, *J. Appl. Physiol. 17:*9 (1962).
49. Sankey, R., Watson, D. *et al.*, Left ventricular function and shunt flow by $C^{15}O_2$ inhalation, *Radiology* (1976).
50. Lederer, C. M., Hollander, J. M., and Perlman, I., *Table of Isotopes,* Sixth Ed., John Wiley & Sons, New York (1968).

PART II • Shunt Detection in Congenital Heart Disease

Scintiangiographic and Probe Systems in the Detection of Cardiac Shunts

William L. Ashburn

Introduction

Radionuclide angiography has been used in the evaluation of pediatric patients with suspected congenital heart disorders for almost seven years.[1-4] The procedure derives its popularity by virtue of requiring nothing more arduous than an intravenous injection of a bolus of ^{99m}Tc pertechnetate (a physiologically inactive agent), followed by imaging with a scintillation camera. This extremely safe and relatively simple technique, which is associated with a comparatively low radiation-absorbed dose, shows promise in screening children with heart murmurs of undetermined etiology or patients with suspicious chest radiographs prior to deciding on the necessity of cardiac catheterization. This essentially noninvasive test can be of particular value in differentiating between hemodynamically insignificant murmurs and murmurs resulting from left-to-right shunts that may necessitate catheterization, a procedure that, in addition to being associated with a certain risk, is considerably more expensive. Radionuclide angiography can be useful on occasion in evaluating neonates in whom it may be difficult to differentiate between primary pulmonary disorders and congenital heart defects. Furthermore, because of the simplicity of the technique, children can be followed after various surgical corrective procedures without requiring frequent repeat catheterizations to evaluate their postoperative status

WILLIAM L. ASHBURN · Division of Nuclear Medicine, Department of Radiology, University of California, San Diego Medical Center, San Diego, California.

With current instrumentation, we can recognize, even in small children, altered patterns in bolus transit through the central circulatory system in various types of congenital heart disease.The intriguing feature of radionuclide angiography, however, is not so much that we can visualize these defects by serial imaging, but that we can express these abnormal relationships (such as the magnitude of a left-to-right shunt) in quantitative or semiquantitative terms by applying sometimes simple, but occasionally more complex, analytical methods.

Before describing these methods, we should examine the injection techniques, since their importance is often overlooked. For quite some time we were convinced that the only way to ensure that the radioactive bolus would arrive centrally without fragmentation or holdup at the thoracic inlet was by inserting a central venous catheter to the level of the superior vena cava.[5] While not too difficult in an adult, it proved to be quite impractical in children.

Our current practice is to inject a small bolus of ^{99m}Tc pertechnetate (approximately 200 μCi/kg) through a 23-g butterfly needle into the external jugular vein (occasionally the femoral vein) and flush this with approximately 2 ml heparinized saline. Since the volume is usually less than 0.5 ml, it is frequently placed within the plastic connection tube and then flushed into the central circulation with one continuous motion without the complicated manipulations of a three-way valve.

As further assurance of an intact bolus, we usually insist on sedation of a young child with an intramuscular "cocktail" of meperidine and promethazine hydrochloride. We have discovered that, all too frequently, an apprehensive or crying child will perform a Valsalva maneuver at the moment of injection and fragment the bolus or trap a portion of it at the thoracic inlet to a degree where only the more gross anatomical features can be appreciated and quantitative measurements are virtually impossible.

Another argument for extreme care in the injection technique is that by maintaining an intact bolus, we maximize the available photon flux emitted from the individual chambers during any 1-sec image frame, which in turn affords improved resolution of that chamber, while at the same time allowing us to lower the injection dose. Indeed, we have observed excellent quality studies in adults with as little as 8–10 mCi ^{99m}TcO$_4^-$ injected into the external jugular vein or through a central venous catheter.

When the bolus is intact, we can recognize certain anatomic features quite clearly on serial 1-sec exposures made with the scintillation detector placed over the anterior chest wall. In small children, rather than using a parallel-hole collimator, we often substitute a converging collimator to increase resolution (by magnification) with little or no sacrifice in sensitivity. In some situations, the detector is placed in the left anterior oblique position with a slight angulation toward the feet to maximally separate the right and the left heart chambers.

In a normal example (Figure 1) in which 2 mCi of $^{99m}TcO_4^-$ were injected into the femoral vein of a small child, we can appreciate that the bolus remained intact on initial arrival (A), and within 1 sec had virtually cleared from the inferior vena cava (B). Furthermore, the bolus arrived in each vascular structure in the correct sequence, i.e., right heart chambers, pulmonary artery, lungs, left heart chambers, aorta, and so on. We also noted how quickly the radioactivity disappeared from the lung fields (i.e., between C and E).

By contrast, what commonly occurs in cases of large left-to-right shunts is shown in Figure 2, row A, in which a portion of the bolus passed through the defect and then reappeared in the lungs, the net effect being prolonged accumulation of radioactivity within the lungs.

Just the opposite is observed (Figure 2, row B) in the case of a Tetralogy of Fallot (right-to-left shunt), in which the abnormal pattern of bolus transit is recognized by the premature appearance of radioactivity in the aorta as well as by markedly diminished activity in both lung fields.

While we may have relatively little difficulty in demonstrating large cardiac shunts by serial imaging as in these examples, this method alone does not allow us to detect small left-to-right shunts nor to quantitate them.

One of the earliest attempts at detecting left-to-right shunts by a radioisotopic-dilution technique was reported in 1962 by Folse and Braunwald.[6] These investigators described a technique for obtaining pulmonary dilution curves following the femoral vein injection of ^{131}I-labeled diodrast and using a single-probe detector that was placed over a region of the patient's chest thought to represent peripheral lung vasculature. They used a strip-chart recorder to plot the appearance and the disappearance of the radionuclide beneath the detector. The resulting dilution curve represented the time vs. concentration relationship of radionuclide while passing through the pulmonary vascular bed beneath the probe, which is somewhat analogous to the indicator-dilution curves obtained during cardiac catheterization.

According to this method, two points (C_1 and C_2) on the curve are defined (Figure 3): Point C_1 corresponds to the maximum counting rate following the initial rise of the curve, and C_2 represents a point on the downslope of the curve occurring at time T_2. Time period T_2 is equal to time T_1, which in turn represents the time between the point at which the count rate begins to exceed background and the point of maximum count rate (C_1). The ratio of the two count rates (C_2/C_1) is then expressed as a percentage.

In about 1969, we applied the same C_2/C_1 technique in evaluating children undergoing radionuclide angiography. All that was required, in addition to a scintillation camera, was some means of data-recording and the facility to assign regions of interest (ROIs) that corresponded to the lung fields to obtain pulmonary dilution curves similar to those produced by a single probe placed over one

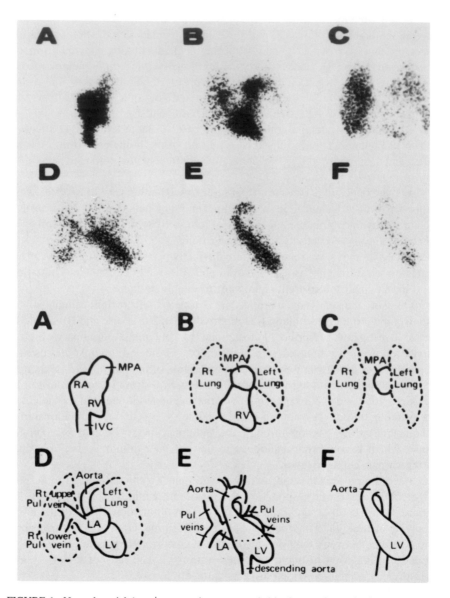

FIGURE 1. Normal, serial 1 sec/exposure images recorded in the anterior projection. Injection of 2/mCi of ^{99m}Tc pertechnetate was made into the femoral vein in a child. The relatively greater concentration of radioactivity in the right lung (C) is not an uncommon finding. (IVC) Inferior vena cava; (MPA) main pulmonary artery; (RA) right atrium; (RV) right ventricle; (LV) left ventricle; (LA) left atrium.

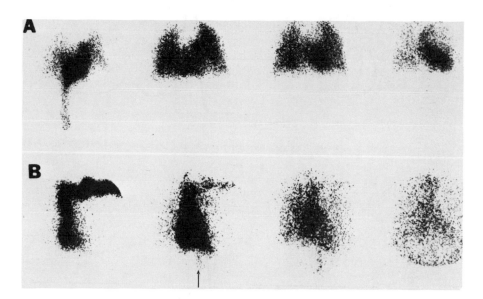

FIGURE 2. Row A—Serial, 1-sec/exposure anterior images in a patient with a left-to-right shunt through a ventricular septal defect. Injection was made into the femoral vein. Note the prolonged clearance of radioactivity from the lungs (fourth image from the left) in comparison with the normal patient (see Figure 1, E); Row B—Patient with a right-to-left shunt (Tetralogy of Fallot). Serial 1-sec images show early appearance of the aorta (arrow) and diminished radioactivity in the lungs. Injection was made into a left peripheral arm vein, and demonstrates a relatively protracted bolus entry into the heart.

or both lung fields. Accordingly, using the scintillation camera and imaging over the heart and lungs, we examined a large series of both normal patients and patients with left-to-right shunts. Regions of interest were placed over one or both lung fields, being careful to avoid any portion of the heart or great vessels within the ROIs. With the aid of a digital computer or analogue data-processing system, which allows assignment of regions of interest corresponding to the lungs, plots of counts appearing within the defined regions against time were generated. C_2/C_1 ratios of less than 32% were consistently calculated in normal patients. In all patients with left-to-right shunts, the C_2/C_1 ratios were greater than 35%. Our results in 93 patients are shown in Figure 4, in which nearly half the patients underwent cardiac catheterization for confirmation of the presence or absence of a left-to-right shunt.[7] The remaining patients were classified as either having shunts or not having shunts on the basis of clinical, radiographic, electrocardiographic, or phonocardiographic data. The patients ranged in age from 2 days to 34 years, with 90% under the age of 18 and half under the age of 5.

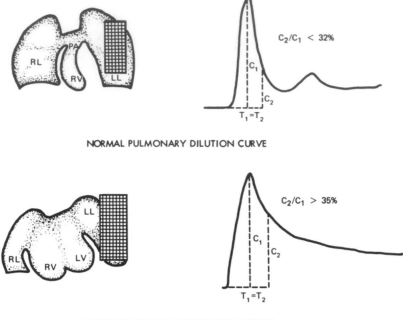

NORMAL PULMONARY DILUTION CURVE

ABNORMAL PULMONARY DILUTION CURVE

LEFT-TO-RIGHT SHUNT

FIGURE 3. Pulmonary dilution curves redrawn from a patient without a cardiac shunt (top row) and one with a left-to-right shunt (bottom row). See the text for the derivation of the C_2/C_1 ratio. (From Alazraki, N. P., Ashburn, W. L., Hagan, A. and Friedman, W. F., Detection of left-to-right shunts with a scintillation camera pulmonary dilution curve, *J. Nucl. Med. 13:*142–147, 1972.)

Patients with left-to-right shunts showed a range of C_2/C_1 ratios between 35 and 96%, with an average of 57%. Seven of the patients with abnormal C_2/C_1 values who underwent cardiac catheterization had small left-to-right shunts detected by hydrogen probe only.

Recent experience has suggested that our detection of accuracy is quite high for shunts that are larger than 1.2:1, but smaller shunts are very difficult to detect. False-positive results do occur but can most often be traced to a poor injection technique (i.e., a fractionated bolus). It should be remembered that other conditions resulting in impaired right ventricular function can be associated with an abnormal C_2/C_1 ratio.[8,9] These can, however, often be excluded on clinical grounds in most cases in which the procedure might otherwise be employed in the screening of patients with suspected left-to-right shunts.

An attempt was made to quantitate the degree of left-to-right shunting by the

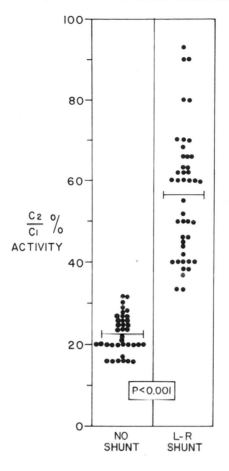

FIGURE 4. C_2/C_1 ratios in 93 patients with and without left-to-right shunts. Patients with other forms of congenital heart disease were excluded. (From Hagan, A. D., Friedman, W. F., Of scintillation scanning techniques in the diagnosis and management of infants and children with congenital heart disease, *Circulation* 45:858–868, 1972.)

C_2/C_1 ratio.[10] Although there was some correlation between the C_2/C_1 ratios and the magnitude of the shunt as expressed by the pulmonary-to-systemic-flow (Q_p/Q_s) ratio determined from oximetry data at the time of cardiac catheterization, precise quantitation was not possible using this technique.

Bosnjakovic *et al.*[11] from UCLA have reported their experience in detecting both left-to-right and right-to-left shunts by analyzing radionuclide dilution curves from selected regions of interest corresponding to specific heart chambers (Figure 5). In normal patients, one notes a prompt rise in count rate to a single

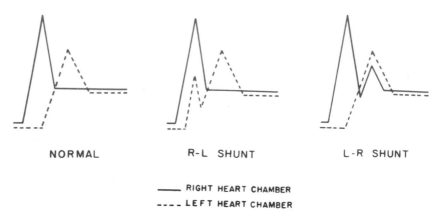

NORMAL   R-L SHUNT   L-R SHUNT

——— RIGHT HEART CHAMBER
– – – – LEFT HEART CHAMBER

FIGURE 5. Typical dilution curves from specific heart chambers. (Redrawn after Bosnjakaovic, V. B., Bennett, L. R., Greenfield, L. D., *et al.,* Dual isotope method for diagnosis of intracardiac shunts, *J. Nucl. Med. 14:*514–521, 1973.)

peak, then a fall toward the baseline, while monitoring both the right and left heart chambers. The right heart peak, of course, appears before the left heart peak. In the case of right-to-left cardiac shunts, a single peak is noted in the right cardiac chamber dilution curve, but an abnormal early peak, corresponding to the blood radioactivity shunted through the defect from right to left, is detected simultaneously from the region of interest corresponding to the left heart chamber. In left-to-right intracardiac shunts, a secondary (shunt) peak is detected over the right heart, representing the shunted radioactive tracer from the left-to-right heart chambers. In theory, if precise placement of the regions of interest can be made to correspond precisely to all or a portion of the atria or ventricles, one should be able to determine the probable site of shunting. In fact, the UCLA group has demonstrated this in several cases of left-to-right shunts at the atrial level and the ventricular level. In the case of atrial septal defects, shunt peaks have been observed only in the right ventricular curve. This is a clever scheme, provided we can accurately identify and separate the right atrium from the right ventricle in radionuclide angiograms, particularly in small children.

In an attempt to quantitate the severity of left-to-right shunts in children, Maltz and Treves[12] at Boston Children's Hospital have suggested a technique to analyze pulmonary dilution curves. A gamma variate is fit to the ascending limb and the first portion of the descending limb of the dilution curve through the use of a small dedicated computer. Based on this derived function, the remainder of the descending limb of the curve is extrapolated downward to the baseline (Figure 6). The area under this curve (Area A) corresponds to the counts obtained during the transit of the radioactive bolus through the pulmonary region of interest without accounting for recirculation through the left-to-right shunt (if

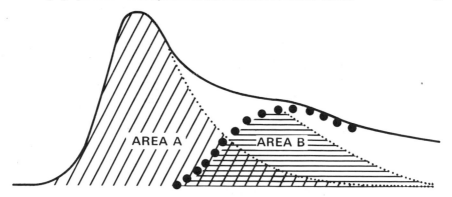

FIGURE 6. Method of Maltz and Treves[12] to calculate pulmonary (Q_p) to systemic (Q_s) flow ratio from a pulmonary dilution curve. The fine dotted line is an extrapolated gamma-variate fit to the pulmonary-dilution curve (continuous line). The point-for-point subtraction of these curves produces a third curve (heavy dots), which is fit with a gamma-variate and extrapolated to the baseline. (See the text for calculation of Q_p/Q_s.)

present). The extrapolated curve is then subtracted point for point from the original dilution curve, which results in a second curve that is, in turn, fit with a gamma variate. This results in a third curve, the area (Area B) under which is proportional to the recirculation of a portion of the radioactive bolus through the left-to-right shunt and again into the pulmonary region of interest. The difference between Area A and Area B provides a number that is proportional to the systemic flow (Q_s). The ratio of pulmonary blood flow to systemic blood flow (Q_p/Q_s) is calculated by dividing area A by the difference between Area A and Area B. Maltz and Treves have shown that Q_p/Q_s ratios can be accurately determined when they fall between 1.2:1 and 3:1. They found an excellent correlation between Q_p/Q_s values determined by oximetry obtained at the time of cardiac catheterization and Q_p/Q_s as determined by the gamma-variate radionuclide method. This method is currently in use in a number of laboratories in which small dedicated computer systems are used to perform the computation.

Another interesting technique has been reported by Weber et al.[13] using a scintillation camera interfaced with a small digital computer. These investigators have described a method of detecting and quantitating right-to-left shunts by analyzing the dilution curves derived from specific cardiac chambers (e.g., RV or LV) in a way that is very similar to the technique used in quantitating Q_p/Q_s proposed by Maltz and Treves. However, they used a more traditional monoexponential fit to the downslope of the dilution curves, rather than employing a gamma-variate fit to the pulmonary-dilution curve. Just as in the case of the method of Bosnjakovic et al.,[11] the accuracy of this technique would appear to be only as good as one's ability to accurately identify and isolate specific heart chambers for the selection of regions of interest.

Summary

The use of radionuclide angiography for intracardiac shunt detection and quantitation is relatively new, and additional patient studies will be needed to accumulate a reliable experience with these methods. Even so, it appears that radionuclide angiography may prove to be an excellent simple screening procedure for patients in the pediatric age group with heart murmurs of undetermined etiology, as well as a tool for following pre- and postoperative shunt patients.

References

1. Mason, D. T., Ashburn, W. L., Harbert, J. C., *et al.*, Rapid visualization of the heart and great vessels in man using the wide-field Anger scintillation camera, radioisotope-angiography following the injection of technetium-99m, *Circulation 39:*19–28 (1968).
2. Burke, G., Halko, A., and Goldberg, D., Dynamic clinical studies with radioisotopes and the scintillation camera. IV. ^{99m}Tc-sodium pertechnetate cardiac blood flow studies, *J. Nucl. Med. 10:*270–280 (1969).
3. Hagan, A. D., Friedman, W. F., Ashburn, W. L., *et al.*, Further applications of scintillation scanning techniques to the diagnosis and management of infants and children with congenital heart disease, *Circulation 45:*858–867 (1972).
4. Hayden, W. G., and Kriss, J. P., Scintiphotographic studies of acquired cardiovascular disease, *Semin. Nucl. Med. 3:*177–190 (1973).
5. Ashburn, W. L., and Braunwald, E., Diagnosis of congenital heart disease, in: *Nuclear Medicine* (2nd Ed.) (William H. Blahd, ed.) McGraw Hill Book Co., New York (1971) pp. 500–513.
6. Folse, R., and Braunwald, E., Pulmonary vascular dilution curves recorded by external detection—the diagnosis of left-to-right shunts, *Brit. Heart. J. 24:*166–172 (1962).
7. Alazraki, N. P., Ashburn, W. L., Hagan, A. D., and Friedman, W. F., Detection of left-to-right shunts with the scintillation camera pulmonary dilution curve, *J. Nucl. Med. 13:*142–147 (1972).
8. Rosenthall, L., Nucleographic screening of patients for left-to-right cardiac shunts, *Radiology 99:*601–604 (1972).
9. Greenfield, L. D., and Bennett, L. R., Comparison of heart chamber and pulmonary dilution curves for diagnosis of cardiac shunts, *Radiology 111:*359–363 (1974).
10. Hagen, A. D., Friedman, W. E., Ashburn, W. L., and Alazraki, N. P., Further applications of scintillation scanning techniques to the diagnosis and management of infants and children with congenital heart disease, *Circulation 45:*858–868 (1972).
11. Bosnjakovic, V. B., Bennett, L. R., Greenfield, L. D., *et al.*, Dual isotope method for diagnosis of intracardiac shunts, *J. Nucl. Med. 14:*514–521 (1973).
12. Maltz, D. L., and Treves, S., Quantitative radionuclide angiography; determination of $Q_p : Q_s$ in children, *Circulation 47:*1049–1056 (1973).
13. Weber, P. M., Dos Remedios, L. V., and Jasko, I. A., Quantitative radioisotopic angiocardiography, *J. Nucl. Med. 13:*815–822 (1972).

Detection of Left-to-Right Shunts by Inhalation of Oxygen-15-Labeled Carbon Dioxide

D. D. Watson, P. J. Kenny, W. R. Janowitz,
D. M. Tamer, and A. J. Gilson

Introduction

The general properties of ^{15}O-labeled carbon dioxide have been reviewed[1,2] and published.[3] The most striking property of this gas is that, when inhaled, it causes the sudden labeling of pulmonary venous blood water and, subsequently, a mathematically predictable clearance from the lungs into the left heart. This property, as we will see, can be most useful in the detection and quantitation of left-to-right intracardiac shunts. We will outline the general methods of shunt detection and quantitation here, and with this as background, a method utilizing the special properties of $C^{15}O_2$ inhalation will be developed and demonstrated.

Detection of Left-to-Right Shunts

The general indicator-dilution principles for detection of left-to-right shunts can be illustrated using the schematic diagram of Figure 1. In this figure, the dotted line shows a shunt flow from the left ventricle (LV) to the right ventricle (RV) for the purpose of illustration, but the basic principles are the same regard-

D. D. WATSON, P. J. KENNY, W. R. JANOWITZ, D. M. TAMER, and A. J. GILSON · University of Miami School of Medicine, Baumritter Institute of Nuclear Medicine, Mount Sinai Medical Center, Miami Beach, Florida.

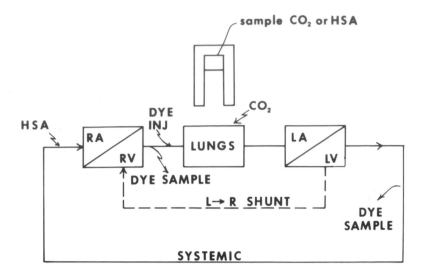

FIGURE 1. Schematic diagram of the central circulation, indicating various points of injection and sampling of indicators for left-to-right shunt detection.

less of the type of shunt. A conventional dye-dilution study performed at catheterization uses the injection of green dye into the pulmonary artery, with sampling of the systemic arterial blood, and indicates a left-to-right shunt by a "break," or abnormal upward deviation, of the downstroke of the dye-dilution curve caused by early recirculation through the shunt pathway. This is characteristic of any method that uses proximal (upstream) injection and distal (downstream) sampling. A much more sensitive and definitive indication of left-to-right shunt flow can be achieved by simultaneous sampling upstream from the point of injection. For example, by injecting dye into the distal right pulmonary artery and sampling in the proximal main pulmonary artery, even the most minute quantity of dye that appears at the sampling site prior to systemic recirculation gives positive indication of a shunt. The same advantage can be obtained by sampling within the right heart or the main pulmonary artery for early traces of hydrogen gas or a radionuclide-labeled gas, such as krypton-85,[4] which can be introduced by inhalation. Again, in this case the sampling site is upstream from the injection site, and the detection threshold is consequently very low due to the absence of background from the normal circulation of the indicator.

Noninvasive methods require the use of radionuclide-labeled indicators that can be sampled with precordial gamma-ray detectors.[5] The lungs are usually chosen as the best sampling site, since this alleviates the problems of measuring activity from a selected heart chamber or great vessel in the presence of interfering activity from adjacent chambers. The injection sites for noninvasive methods must then be either peripheral veins or radionuclide-labeled gases administered by inhalation. ^{15}O-Labeled CO_2 is an ideal substance for inhalation because of the properties discussed previously. A unique feature of this technique is that the lung fields then become both the site of injection as well as the site of sampling. The detection threshold for this technique will therefore tend to be intermediate between the highest sensitivity, which can be achieved by sampling proximal to the injection site, and the lower sensitivity, which is achieved in sampling distal to the injection site. In this case, the methods for both detection and quantitation are similar to other indicator-dilution methods, but will differ in detail to accommodate the particular injection and sampling site.

Quantitation of Left-to-Right Shunts

All radionuclide methods for shunt determination are based on the indicator-dilution principle of sampling the concentration of a bolus injection as the bolus passes a sampling point in the central circulation. However, indicator-dilution measurements, although performed, are not used to quantitate shunts in current cardiac catheterization practice. The Fick method, applied to oxygen concentration (oximetry), is the presently accepted quantitative standard, and will therefore be reviewed for the purpose of comparison. By oximetry, the pulmonary-to-systemic-flow ratio Q_p/Q_s can be expressed as

$$Q_p/Q_s = \frac{C_a - C_v}{C_a - C_p}$$

where C_a and C_v are, respectively, the systemic arterial and venous oxygen concentrations, and C_p is the oxygen concentration obtained from pulmonary arterial blood or from a mixed blood sample taken between the shunt site and the lungs. The shunt flow, expressed as a function f of pulmonary flow, is

$$f = \frac{C_p - C_v}{C_a - C_v}$$

Since this measurement is made at equilibrium, there are no problems associated with an indicator bolus or with recirculation. The principal source of potential error is in obtaining blood samples in which the various components of systemic venous blood and/or blood from shunt flow are not completely and uniformly mixed. This technique can, of course, only be performed invasively

The indicator-dilution method used in noninvasive measurements requires the analysis of an indicator-dilution (ID) curve following a bolus injection. Shunt quantitation can be obtained by knowing the area A under the curve, which

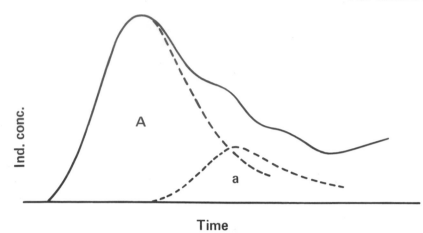

FIGURE 2. Indicator-dilution curve with shunt recirculation, showing the decomposition into primary circulation and shunt recirculation components. The relative areas of these two curve components are required for shunt quantitation.

includes only the primary bolus transit, relative to the area a under the portion of the curve, caused only by the first shunt recirculation, as indicated in Figure 2 and also discussed by Ashburn.[5] The shunt is calculated by

$$Q_p/Q_s = \frac{A}{A-a}$$

or

$$f = \frac{a}{A}$$

The main problems presented by this technique are the integrity of the bolus and the separation of the curve components corresponding to primary circulation, shunt recirculation, systemic recirculation, multiple-shunt recirculation, and background from systemic circulation. This problem is illustrated by Figure 3, in which the measured ID curve is decomposed in three different ways, yielding widely disparate values for Q_p/Q_s. The problem is further complicated by the fact that as the initial bolus travels from the point of injection, it is dispersed and diluted through successive mixing chambers, becoming progressively spread out and reduced in amplitude. Figure 4 shows calculated ID-curve shapes as they would appear when sampled progressively downstream from the site of injection. When shunt recirculation occurs, the shunt recirculation component has necessarily passed through more mixing chambers than the primary circulation component detected at the same sampling point, and this must be properly accounted for to obtain correct results.

The most simple and widely used analytic method which is applicable to upstream intravenous injections of radionuclide indicators is the C_2/C_1-ratio method (Figure 5) developed by Wood[6] and discussed by Ashburn.[5] The validity of this method rests on the implicit assumptions that the peak of the shunt recirculation component of the ID curve is related to the build-up time of the primary circulation component, and that the relative curve areas are linearly related to the relative curve amplitudes. These assumptions can be approximately justified within the context of a conventional mathematical model of the central circulation. The C_2/C_1-ratio method is thus more rigorous and elegant than would appear from the extreme simplicity of its application. The implicit assumptions, and thus the accuracy of this method, break down when the ID-curve shapes are distorted from their normal shape due to problems with the bolus introduction or hemodynamic abnormalities, such as valvular insufficiency and ventricular failure. In these cases, the downstroke segment of the ID curve will be abnormally elevated and produce an elevated C_2/C_1 ratio even though no shunt is present, giving the potential for a false-positive shunt indication. Also, the differentiation between a "normal" and an "abnormal" C_2/C_1 ratio must be made on the basis of comparing the results from the patient under study to the average value obtained from patients known not to have shunts. It is thus a relative measurement as compared to an absolute measurement, such as oximetry.

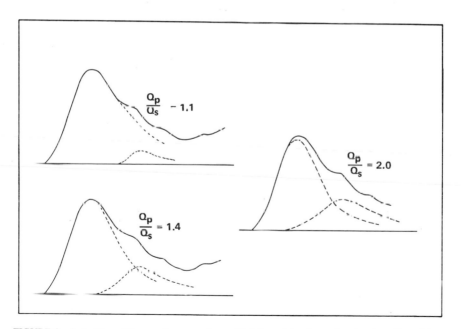

FIGURE 3. Actual lung ID curve from a patient with left-to-right shunt, showing the effect of three alternative ways of decomposing the compound curve.

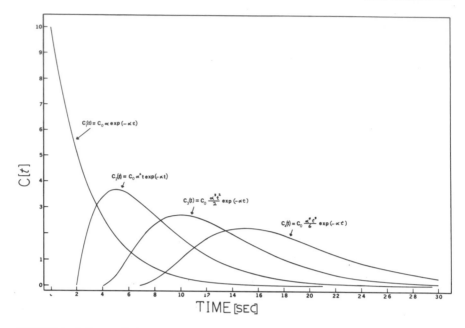

FIGURE 4. Indicator-dilution curve shapes obtained from sampling the same bolus injection at successive chambers downstream from the point of injection.

A second analytic method uses computer-curve fitting of gamma-variate functions to separate the primary and shunt recirculation components of the ID curve.[7] This technique is apparently much more sophisticated mathematically, but it will be subject to some of the same potential sources of error. In clinical applications, the reliability and accuracy of these two methods would probably depend heavily on the injection technique, patient population and controls, skill, and judgment in performing the study and interpreting the results.

The method for quantitation of data from $C^{15}O_2$ inhalation studies has been adapted to the situation where injection and sampling both occur in the lungs. The important consequence of this method is that the lung clearance rate will be precisely monoexponential initially. This is not due to the physiologic process in the lungs, but is the general statistical property for the rate of removal of an indicator from its point of injection. By using a monoexponential extrapolation of the initial downslope segment of the lung clearance curve, we are thus able to separate the primary circulation component of the ID curve completely and correctly.

The system is represented schematically by Figure 6. An indicator-dilution model, including multiple-shunt recirculation, has been used, it expresses the

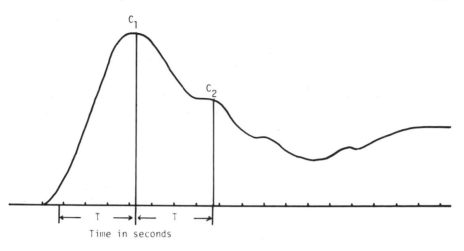

FIGURE 5. Shunt ID curve demonstrating the C_2/C_1-ratio method of analysis.

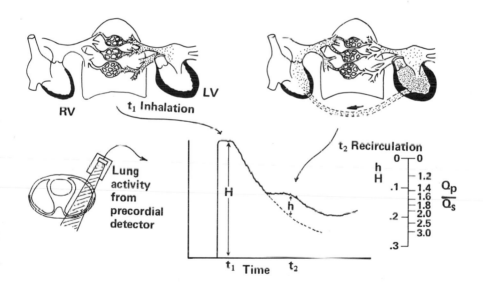

FIGURE 6. Simplified representation of the cardiopulmonary system demonstrating the principle of left-to-right shunt detection by $C^{15}O_2$ inhalation. Early recirculation of tracer into lung fields indicates the existence of a left-to-right shunt.

functional form of the lung-sampled ID curve as

$$C(t) = C_0 \sum_{n=1}^{\infty} \frac{\alpha^n}{(n-1)!} (t - n\Delta)^{n-1} e^{-\alpha(t-n\Delta)}$$

where α is the lung clearance coefficient, f is the shunt flow as a fraction of pulmonary flow, and Δ is the shunt reappearance delay time. A remarkably simple expression for shunt flow which has been derived from this is

$$f = e \ (h/H)$$

where e is 2.72 (base of natural logs), H is the amplitude of the lung clearance curve at the time of inspiration, and h is the amplitude of the peak shunt recirculation measured from the extrapolated initial clearance curve as a baseline. This technique for quantitation is illustrated in Figure 7. The pulmonary-to-systemic-flow ratio is expressed as

$$Q_p/Q_s = \frac{1}{1 - e(h/H)}$$

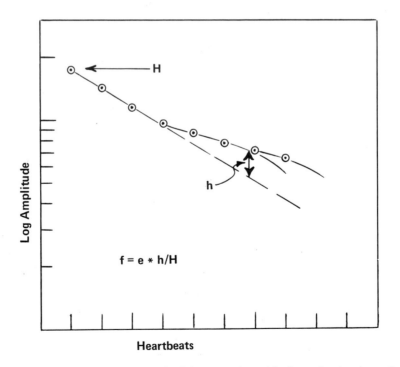

FIGURE 7. Lung clearance curve obtained from a patient with shunt, showing the method of calculating the shunt fraction f from the $C^{15}O_2$ study.

The formalism implies the assumption that curve area ratios can be related to curve amplitude ratios by using the theoretically calculated factor $e = 2.72$. Discussion of the theoretical justification for this assumption will be deferred, but the results of experimental comparative studies that support the validity of this analytic technique will be included. As shown in Figure 7, this method uses the observed primary lung clearance as a baseline and measures the shunt recirculation relative to that baseline. The calculation is absolute in that it is not based on any relative comparison to a "normal" lung clearance rate. Thus, the shunt flow can be quantitated in the presence of concomitant factors, such as valvular insufficiency or ventricular failure, that cause delayed clearance from the lungs.

This method is specific to the inhalation technique and cannot be directly applied to ID data obtained from intravenous injections. In those cases the primary lung clearance is not exponential, and, more importantly, the conversion factor e would be quite incorrect. A different factor is required for each specific point of injection and sampling.

Inhalation Studies

The methods of production and administration of $C^{15}O_2$ and the instrumentation and examples of results have been discussed.[1] Detection probes are placed over the heart and lungs, and a bolus of 5–10 cc labeled CO_2 is introduced into the airway as the patient takes a normal tidal-volume breath. Breath-holding is requested in cooperative patients; however, the transfer of oxygen-15 to pulmonary blood occurs so rapidly that it will be complete before expiration even at the highest possible respiratory rates, and breathing does not significantly interfere with the test. Test results are obtained immediately and can be repeated within the same time needed to produce another gas bolus (about 5 min). Figure 8 shows the complete test results obtained from a normal young adult; Figure 9 shows the test results from a child proved to have an innocent murmur. When analyzed as described, this study can definitively rule out the presence of a left-to-right shunt.

A prospective double-blind study is currently in progress to evaluate the inhalation study for the measurement of left-to-right intracardiac shunts. Table 1 summarizes the results from 24 patients (ages 2–16) who were admitted for elective cardiac catheterization. Figure 10 shows the semilog plots of the lung clearance curves from the first 3 patients of this series. When the lung clearance curve does not show a clearly visible break from a straight line on the semilog plot, as with patient 3 in Figure 10, the test is taken as negative for the presence of a left-to-right shunt. In this series, 9 patients had no evidence of a left-to-right shunt at the time of cardiac catheterization by oximetry or angiography, of this group, 8 had shunt-flow values of exactly zero by inhalation, and 1 had a visible deviation in the lung clearance curve corresponding to a shunt fraction of 5%. This finding was interpreted as negative. In general, any indications for shunts

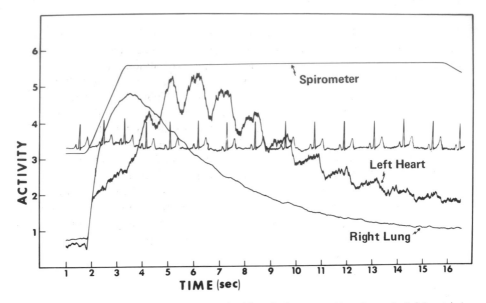

FIGURE 8. Activity–time curve for a normal subject. Probes are positioned over the left heart and the right lung as indicated. The spirometer trace indicates the breathing maneuver, and the ECG signal is also recorded.

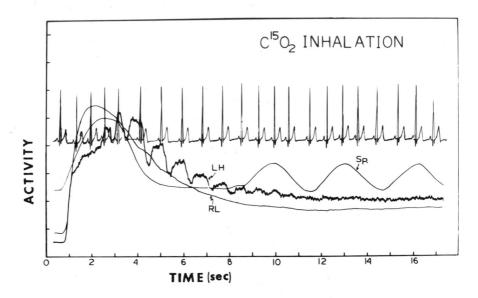

FIGURE 9. Inhalation study of a child found to have an innocent murmur. The spirometer trace indicates that the child was not breath-holding, but nevertheless the lung clearance curve is monoexponential, with no indication of shunt flow. Ejection from the heart is very rapid, suggesting hyperdynamic flow as the cause of the murmur.

TABLE 1. Percentage Values of Left-to-Right Shunt
Flow As Determined by $C^{15}O_2$ Inhalation Technique
and by Oximetry at Catheterization on a Series
of Patients

Patient	$C^{15}O_2$	Oximetry	Diagnosis[a]
1	47	38	VSD
2	23	29	VSD[b]
3	0	0	AS
4	38	69	ASD
5	0	0	AS
6	67	63	ASD
7	67	60	VSD
8	0	0	AS
9	0	0	Postop[c]
10	41	47	ASD
11	38	38	VSD
12	39	44	PAPVR
13	22	29	VSD
14	50	52	ASD
15	5	0	COA
16	0	0	PFO
17	24	0	VSD[d]
18	0	0	PS
19	22	29	VSD
20	0	0	COA
21	23	23	VSD
22	65	50	VSD
23	0	0	AS
24	39	47	ASD

[a](AS) Aortic stenosis; (ASD) atrial septal defect, (VSD) ventricular septal defect; (PAPVR) partial anomalous pulmonary
venous return; (PFO) patent foramen ovale; (PS) pulmonary
stenosis; (COA) coarctation of aorta.
[b]Bidirectional.
[c]VSD, surgically closed.
[d]Negative by oximetry, but VSD confirmed by cineangiography.

less than 10% are interpreted as negative, and only indications greater than 20%
are interpreted as positive. On this basis, the inhalation test results were in
complete agreement with the classifications by catheterization. These results are
indicated in Figure 11. The quantitative agreement is indicated in Figure 12.

The shunt-flow values from the CO_2 studies are absolute values obtained
from the derived formula and have not been adjusted by regression coefficients.
Similarly, the solid line in Figure 12 is the line of identity and not a regression
line. The Pearson r coefficient for all the data is 0.94; the RMS deviation of the
CO_2 values is ±10% from the percentage values obtained by oximetry. Since
some portion of these errors must be due to the oximetry measurements, we

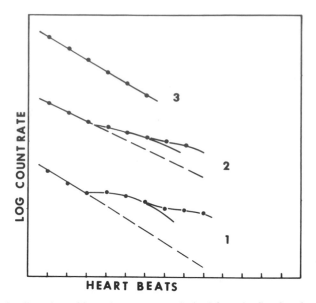

FIGURE 10. Semilog plots of lung clearance rates obtained from the first 3 patients of the shunt study summarized in Table 1.

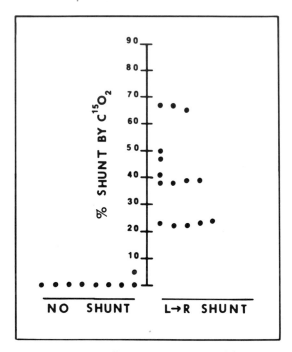

FIGURE 11. Values obtained by the $C^{15}O_2$ inhalation test for left-to-right shunts. Left—patients found to have no shunt at catheterization. Right—patients with documented shunts.

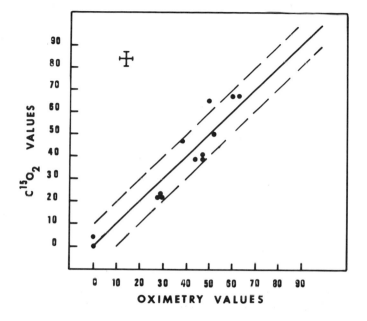

FIGURE 12. Comparison of values for left-to-right shunts, as measured by the $C^{15}O_2$ inhalation test and by oximetry at catheterization. Point 0 represents 9 patients. The solid line is the line of identity; the dashed lines are ±10% from the identity line.

may tentatively conclude from these preliminary data that the errors from the CO_2 inhalation are roughly comparable to the errors expected from oximetry.

Discussion

Radionuclide methods for shunt determinations have been extensively studied.[8-32] Probably the most important and certainly the most neglected problem with conventional methods has been the requirement to achieve a true bolus input to the right heart. Dr. Ashburn has made an important contribution to the solution of this problem. A second problem is in the quantitation of indicator-dilution studies obtained from upstream injections. We are still far from having an entirely satisfactory method to solve this problem, even with computer techniques.

The $C^{15}O_2$ inhalation technique obviates both problems, and consequently may provide greater reliability and accuracy. Correct shunt quantitation is obtained even in the presence of valvular insufficiency or ventricular failure. The test is remarkably simple and rapid, entirely noninvasive, and thus generally well accepted by nonsedated children. The disadvantage is, of course, the lack of general availability of $C^{15}O_2$. However, we are confident that as more new applications for the C, N, and O radioisotopes become known, future developments will bring these isotopes into general availability.

References

1. Kenny, P. J., Watson, D. D., Janowitz, W. R., and Gilson, A. J., The use of $C^{15}O_2$ in the evaluation of cardiac abnormalities, in: *Cardiovascular Investigation with Radionuclides,* Plenum Press, New York (1976).
2. Nickles, R. J., Nelson, P. J., Polcyn, R. E., *et al.,* Radioactive gases in the evaluation of ventricular function, in: *Cardiovascular Investigation with Radionuclides,* Plenum Press, New York (1976).
3. Watson, D. D., Kenny, P. J., Gelband, H., *et al.,* A noninvasive technique for the study of cardiac hemodynamics utilizing $C^{15}O_2$ inhalation, *Radiology 119:*615–622 (June 1976).
4. Braunwald, E., Goldblatt, A., Long, R., and Morrow, A. G., The krypton-85 inhalation test for the detection of left-to-right shunts, *Br. Heart J. 33:*47–54 (1961).
5. Ashburn, W. L., Scintiangiographic and probe systems in the detection of cardiac shunts, in: *Cardiovascular Investigation with Radionuclides,* Plenum Press, New York (1976).
6. Carter, S. A., Bajee, D. F., Yannicelli, E., and Wood, E. H., Estimation of left-to-right shunt from arterial dilution curves, *J. Lab. Clin. Med. 55:*77–88, (Jan. 1960).
7. Maltz, D. L., and Treves, S., Quantitative radionuclide angiography, *Circulation 47:*1049–1056 (1973).
8. Prinzmetal, M., Corday, E., and Spritzler, R. S., Radiocardiography and its clinical applications, *J. Amer. Med. Assoc. 10:*617 (1949).
9. Braunwald, E., Pfaff, E. W., Long, R. T. L., and Morrow, A. G., A simplified indicator dilution technic for the localization of the left-to-right circulatory shunts, *Circ. 20:*875 (1959).
10. Greenspan, R. H., Lester, R. G., Marvin, J. F., and Amplatz, K., Isotope circulation studies in congenital heart disease, *J. Amer. Med. Assoc. 169:*667 (1959).
11. Turner, J. D., Salazar, E., and Gorlin, R., Detection of intracardiac shunts by an external surface counting technic, *Amer. J. Cardiol. 6:*1004 (1960).
12. Shapiro, W., and Sharpe, A. R., Precordial isotope-dilution curves in congenital heart disease: a simple method for the detection of intracardiac shunts, *Amer. Heart J. 60:*607 (1960).
13. Cornell, W. P., Braunwald, E., and Morrow, A. F., Precordial scanning: Application in the detection of left-to-right circulatory shunts, *Circulation 23:*21 (1961).
14. Clarke, J. M., Deegan, T., McKendrick, C. S., Berbert, R. J. T., and Kulke, W., Technetium-99*m* in the diagnosis of left-to-right shunts, *Thorax 21:*79 (1966).
15. Folse, R., and Braunwald, E., Pulmonary vascular dilution curves recorded by external detection in the diagnosis of left-to-right shunts, *Br. Heart J. 24:*106 (1962).
16. Spach, M. S., Canent, R. V., Boineau, J. P., White, A. W., Sanders, A. P., and Baylin, G. J., Radioisotope-dilution curves as an adjunct to cardiac catheterization. *Amer. J. Cardiol 16:*165 (1965).
17. Flaherty, J., Canent, R., Boineau, J., Anderson, P. A. W., Levin, A. R., and Spach, M. S., Use of externally recorded radioisotope dilution curves for quantitation of left-to-right shunts, *Amer. J. Cardiol 20:*341 (1967).
18. Campione, K. M., and Steiner, S. H., Analysis of precordial isotope dilution curves obtained after antecubital and intracardiac injection, *J. Nucl. Med. 9:*630 (1968).
19. Mason, D. T., Ashburn, W. L., Harbert, J. C., *et al.,* Rapid visualization of the heart and great vessels in man using the wide-field Anger scintillation camera, radioisotope-angiography following the injection of technetium-99*m, Circulation 39:*19–28 (1968).
20. Burke, G., Halko, A., and Goldberg, D., Dynamics clinical studies with radioisotopes and the

scintillation camera. IV. ^{99m}Tc-Sodium pertechnetate cardiac blood flow studies, *J. Nucl. Med. 10:*270–280 (1969).

21. Kinoshita, M., Nakao, K., Yoshitsuga, N., Torizuka, K., and Takayasu, M., Detection of circulatory shunts by means of external counting method, *Jp. Circ. J. 33:*815 (1969).

22. Ashburn, W. L., and Braunwald, E., Diagnosis of congenital heart disease, in: *Nuclear Medicine* (W. H. Blahd, ed.), Second Ed. pp. 500–513, McGraw-Hill Book Co. New York (1971).

23. Wesselhoeft, H., Hurley, P. J., Wagner, H. N., and Rowe, R. D., Nuclear angiocardiography in the diagnosis of congenital heart disease in infants, *Circulation 45:*77 (1972).

24. Bosnjakovic, V., Bennett, L., and Vincent, W., Diagnosis of intracardiac shunts without cardiac catheterization, *Circulation 43* (suppl. II):II-144 (1971).

25. Graham, T. P., Goodrich, J. K., Robinson, A. E., and Harris, C. C., Scintiangiocardiography in children: Rapid sequence visualization of the heart and great vessels after intravenous injection of radionuclide, *Amer. J. Cardiol. 25:*387 (1970).

26. Hagan, A. D., Friedman, W. F., Ashburn, W. C., and Alazraki, N., Further application of scintillation scanning technics to the diagnosis and management of infants and children with congenital heart disease, *Circulation 45:*858 (1972).

27. Kriss, J. P., Enright, L. P., Hayden, W. G., Wexter, L., and Shumway, N. E., Radioisotopic angiocardiography, wide scope of applicability in diagnosis and evaluation of therapy in diseases of the heart and great vessels, *Circulation 43:*792 (1971).

28. Alazraki, N. P., Ashburn, W. L., Hagen, A. D., *et al.,* Detection of left-to-right shunts with the scintillation camera pulmonary dilution curve, *J. Nucl. Med. 13:*142–147 (1972).

29. Rosenthall, L., Nucleographic screening of patients for left-to-right cardiac shunts, *Radiology 99:*601–604 (1972).

30. Weber, P. M., Dos Remedios, L. V., and Jasko, L. A., Quantiative radioisotopic angiocardiography, *J. Nucl. Med. 13:*815–822 (1972).

31. Stocker, F. P., Kinser, J., Weber, J. W., and Rosler, H., Pediatric radiocardioangiography: Shunt diagnosis, *Circulation 47:*819–826 (April 1973).

32. Greenfield, L. D., and Bennett, L. R., Comparison of heart chamber and pulmonary dilution curves for diagnosis of cardiac shunts, *Radiology 111:*359–363 (1974).

Part III · Evaluation of Myocardial Blood Flow and Disease

Myocardial Energetics

Frank J. Hildner

Introduction

Successful imaging of any organ requires a basic knowledge of the physiology of the tissue involved. In considering the heart, it is important to realize that the myocardium is richly vascular at all times, both in the normal resting state and in the chronic postinfarction state. This is particularly true during acute myocardial infarction, when the inflammatory process envelops the area of ischemia, rendering the entire zone plethoric and even hemorrhagic. The changes that occur in the metabolic processes at the time of myocardial injury are important to the physician who wishes to tag these areas with radionuclides. The uptake of compounds is largely dependent on the integrity and nature of existing metabolic processes. It is therefore worthwhile to consider the changes that occur in the myocardium throughout the various stages from normal aerobic metabolism to total infarction and anaerobic metabolism.

Problems with Imaging and Infarct. Myocardial infarctions may be divided into two basic types. The first, *transmural infarctions,* are said to occupy most of the thickness of the wall of the myocardium, frequently including the epicardium. It is not necessary, however, for all layers of the heart at a given point to be involved for the infarct to be termed transmural. The second type, the *subendocardial infarction,* usually is limited to the inner 50% of the cardiac wall, sparing the endocardium, which is usually nourished by the blood in the cavity of the heart. Both infarcts may be multiple and variable in position. It is characteristic, however, for the subendocardial infarction to extend more widely

FRANK J. HILDNER · Department of Medicine, University of Miami School of Medicine, Miami, Florida; Department of Cardiology, Mt. Sinai Medical Center, Miami Beach, Florida.

throughout the inner layers of the heart than an individual transmural. Thus, multiple subendocardial infarctions may underlie viable muscle, whereas a transmural infarction may be superimposed on a subendocardial that is already present. Furthermore, both types of infarctions may be extremely small or massive in any area of the myocardium.[1]

The anatomy of the left ventricle frequently makes imaging of a myocardial infarction difficult.[1] The subendocardial infarction may extend circumferentially around the entire chamber of the heart, but may be visualized only in the lateral extremes of the ventricular wall when the wall is perpendicular to the viewing camera. The area of infarction that is covered by viable tissue may be so poorly tagged that it is virtually invisible[2]; multiple small subendocardial infarctions may be so diffuse that none can be distinguished from surrounding viable tissue.[3] A true, even transmural infarction of the posterior wall, when viewed through the anterior wall, may be largely obscured or invisible. Thus, multiple views of the anterior, medial, lateral, and posterior walls of the myocardium are necessary for complete evaluation.[4] Progressive extended sites of infarction may have characteristics of both acute and chronic ischemia, thereby making imaging with a single agent difficult or impossible.

Another frequently misunderstood concept concerning myocardial infarction deals with the incidence of coronary artery occlusion or thrombosis. Recently, Roberts compiled a list of 3410 patients who sustained acute myocardial infarction. Of this number only 1944 (57%) were shown to have coronary thrombosis.[2] Put another way, 43% did not sustain complete coronary occlusion. These results are not surprising to physicians performing coronary arteriography who are confronted with these findings on a day-to-day basis.[3] It is not uncommon to find subendocardial areas of the left ventricle with small and patchy infarctions leading to segmental myocardial hypokinesis or akinesis due to massive ventricular hypertrophy, secondary to systemic arterial hypertension. Severe coronary sclerosis with severe but nonobstructive disease is also a potential cause. Other diagnoses frequently associated with myocardial infarction and patent coronary vessels include calcific aortic stenosis, valvular aortic insufficiency with severe myocardial hypertrophy, pulmonary embolism, severe acute anemia, occlusion of mesenteric arteries, pulmonary embolism, and operative procedures associated with hypotension and serious electrolyte imbalance.

In those cases with coronary artery occlusion, atherosclerosis is statistically the most common underlying etiology. If the atherosclerotic process is sufficiently diffuse, poor perfusion scanning would be expected.[4] However, if the process were highly localized and most coronary vessels were relatively large and free of occlusion, myocardial perfusion scanning would be essentially normal in all areas. In planning a scan, one should not assume that coronary atherosclerosis is the only process in operation. Where severe myocardial injury has occurred, coronary embolism frequently occurs as repeated infarction.

Embolism may also occur from rheumatic, atrial, or ventricular foci, as well as from rheumatic or prosthetic aortic and mitral valves. Disease processes of the aorta and coronary vessels themselves, such as periarteritis, giant-cell arteritis, and dystrophic calcification of the coronary arteries, have been shown to cause total coronary occlusion. Thrombotic occlusion of the ostia of the coronary arteries is not common. However, clot build up on an aortic-valve prosthesis has been shown frequently to occlude the coronary ostia. Similarly, a dissecting aneurysm of the ascending aortic arch may dissect retrograde to the area of the aortic valve and cause occlusions of either the right or the left coronary vessels.

Tissue Response to Abnormal Blood Flow

Acute Responses to Myocardial Ischemia. No structural change or damage occurs in the myocardium if normal blood supply is reestablished after 5 min of total ischemia or up to 20 min of partial ischemia. Ischemia lasting over 20 min produces focal areas of necrosis, fibrosis, or massive infarction, depending on the oxygen consumption of the individual area. Infarction, however, may occur without total occlusion from many causes (as listed) when oxygen utilization exceeds oxygen supply. Local coronary narrowing produces collateral branches and these occur only if occlusion occurs relatively slowly, i.e., over a period of days, weeks, or months. Some collateral vessels may form within 2 or 3 days, but usually require 12 days for adequate function. Collateral branches of 40 μm size require 2 or 3 weeks of an ischemic stimulus for formation.

The size of an infarction, or area of ischemia, is determined by a host of factors. If a major coronary vessel is occluded proximally, collateral flow from the vessel of the opposite side will frequently prevent massive infarction. However, if occlusion of a medium-sized coronary vessel occurs halfway out its course, no collateral flow may be possible and a large infarct will result. Thus, the size of the occluded artery and the site of the occlusion are major determinants of infarct size. Similarly, complete total occlusion or the rapid development of an ischemic process is more likely to produce a larger severe infarct than a rather slow onset of either process. If the ischemic area is the result of a singular vascular occlusion or insult and other coronary vessels are completely normal, the possibilities of a major infarct are somewhat reduced. Similarly, the anatomic pattern of the coronary vessels and the degree of collateral circulation existent at the time of the ischemic process way heavily on the degree and extent of infarction. With all other factors being equal, severe myocardial hypertrophy, anemia, polycythemia, and similar conditions are important determinants of infarct size.

Anatomical Changes to Acute Ischemia—Infarction. Total ischemia of a given area results in prompt cyanosis with the rapid appearance of pallor.

Discoloration with a brownish mottling occurs macroscopically and may subsequently turn to frank hemorrhage. In 5–10 min, microscopic examination will reveal clumping of the nucleoplasm; cytoplasmic distortion with vacuoles will appear at the same time the mitochondria begin to swell. After 30–40 min, irreversible distortion of the mitochrondrial structures occur; after 8 hr, edema of the interstitial tissues is seen with deposition of large fat droplets. At 24 hr, disruption of nuclei and cell membranes is obvious. Infiltration of polymorphonuclear leukocytes and red blood cells into the interstitial tissues begins and lasts for approximately 1 week. Hyalin and brick-red muscle fibers, devoid of nuclei or striations, appear and ghosts of cells are found. Within 48 hr, fibroblasts begin to appear with lymphocytes and mononuclear cells, peaking at 3 to 4 weeks. Peripheral hemorrhage becomes more prominent at this time and organization begins. At 4 days, healing becomes predominant with many fibroblasts appearing along with granulation tissue and vascular ingrowth. At 2 weeks, healing is virtually complete for small infarcts. However, the hard avascular scar is not complete until 4–5 weeks, when the classic scar is finally formed.

Hemodynamic Changes. In classic experiments by Wiggers,[5] occlusion of a single coronary vessel results in a rapid decrease in contractility, which is soon followed by passive paradoxical motion (outward) in systole with a marked decrease in force and velocity of contraction. The *dP/dt* is reduced, and systemic systolic pressure falls. The systolic ejection rate, cardiac output, and stroke volume soon decrease also. A decreased ejection fraction soon results in a markedly increased end-systolic volume, with delayed peak force appearing systemically. A rapid increase in the left ventricular end-diastolic pressure occurs with simultaneous increases in left-atrial mean pressure and pulmonary artery pressures.

Cellular Structure. Microscopically, the reason for these marked hemodynamic changes is marked destruction of the basic structural building block of the muscle cell, namely, the *sarcomere*.[6] The sarcomere is composed of interdigitating actin and myosin fibers that are called *thick* and *thin bands*. These fibers are nourished by an elaborate system of intercellular channels, called the *T system*, which is part of the sarcoplasmic reticulum supplying both nourishment and a route for conduction of impulses between the muscle cells and the fibers. The basic nutrients for contraction, such as calcium ion, as well as sodium and potassium ion, are supplied through this system. The intracellular site of metabolism providing most of the energy for cardiac metabolism is the mitochondria, which are also located intracellularly. These structures are located within the sarcolemma and have been reported in some instances to account for 25% of the weight of cardiac muscle. Once substrates supplied through the blood reach the mitochondria, high levels of high-energy phosphates, such as ATP (adenosine triphosphate) and CP (creatine phosphate), are formed, which permit cardiac contraction that occurs between the thin and thick filaments of the muscle fibers. Excitation transmitted via the tubular systems through the sarcolemma and the T system results in a depolarization of the cell membrane with a rapid influx of sodium and an outflow of potassium from the cell. The resultant depolarization causes release of calcium within the cell and the entry of extracellular calcium into the sarcoplasm. At this point, contraction occurs by the extremely rapid formation of the bridges between the actin and the myosin fibers, resulting in a physical sliding of the thin fibers between the thick fibers and a decrease in the distance between the Z bands (ends) of the sarcomere. Movement then occurs by the shortening of the sarcomere, resulting from chemical bonds being created between the two filaments. The rapid resolution of these bridges permits the fiber to return to its resting state (with an efflux of calcium from the cell) and the chemical metabolic structure returns to its resting state in anticipation of the next impulse.

Histochemical Changes and Myocardial Energy Sources. Hypoxia rapidly decreases myocardial function, decreasing oxidative phosphorylation, the major source of energy produced as part of the citric acid cycle. At this point the heart shifts from an aerobic metabolism in the mitochondria to an anaerobic glycolysis in the cytoplasm.[7]

The major source of energy utilized by the myocardium for contraction is a result of metabolism that occurs aerobically in the mitochondria. This is the result of metabolism of substrates to high-energy phosphates, which are then converted by the cardiac fibers to external work with the subsequent liberation of carbon dioxide and water. The energetics that occur in the cardiac muscle may be divided into three general categories:

1. *Energy liberation,* which occurs in the citric acid cycle
2. *Energy conservation,* which includes the formation of high-energy phosphate bonds
3. *Energy utilization,* which encompasses the conversion of actin and myosin to actomysin with the conversion of free calcium ion to bound calcium in the subsequent production of cardiac work

Energy Liberation. There are four basic substrates for aerobic myocardial metabolism: free fatty acids; glucose; lactate, pyruvate, and ketone bodies; and amino acids. All four categories enter the citric acid cycle and, after completely traversing the aerobic metabolic pathway, result in 36 high-energy phosphate bonds. This is in distinction to the anaerobic metabolism of glucose that occurs in the cytoplasm of the myocardial cell, which bypasses the citric acid cycle and results in only two high-energy phosphate bonds produced for every molecule metabolized.

Free fatty acids enter the citric acid cycle by hydrolysis, permitting β-oxidation of a two-carbon fragment at the end of each fatty acid chain. This two-carbon fragment enters the citric acid cycle after condensing with acetyl coenzyme A. Glucose, on the other hand, a six-carbon molecule, is first split to a three-carbon fragment, which is then converted to three-carbon lactate or pyruvate, by which it enters the cycle. Ketone bodies, such as β-hydroxybutyric acid or acetone, are converted first to acetoacetic acid, and from there are condensed with the acetyl coenzyme A and enter the citric acid cycle in this form. Amino acids are the least important metabolic substrate but enter the citric acid cycle as oxaloacetic acid after the NH_3 group is acted on by deaminase and oxidized by amino acid oxidase.

Energy Conservation. As electrons are transported through the citric acid cycle and energy is released, this energy is conserved by oxidative phosphorylation. The conversion of ADP to ATP and the intraconversion of ATP and creatine phosphate result in a large pool of high-energy phosphates ready for metabolic demand at the site of utilization. Energy utilization occurs when ATP or CP is hydrolyzed by myofibrillar ATPase to ADP and phosphate.

Recognition of the inherent properties of myocardial tissue permit accurate prediction of which radionuclides may be useful in obtaining satisfactory images. Since potassium is the predominant intracellular ion, one may assume that any nuclide that is recognized by the body, as in the family of potassium ion, and that has basic properties similar to this ion, may be exchanged for potassium and thereby tag that myocardial cell. Of course, ionic potassium itself would be the optimum choice, but its selection is hindered by its high-energy characteristics, making it unsuitable from a technical standpoint. Another major ion present in large quantities in the myocardial cell is phosphate in both free and complex forms. Since large quantities of high- and low-energy phosphate are always present in the myocardium, incorporation of a nuclide that is recognized by the heart as acting like phosphorus or a member of this family would probably provide excellent imaging. Since the heart is extremely vascular, it is unlikely that an attempt at tagging the scar itself would be at all successful. Negative imaging of the scar by heavy incorporation of nuclide in the surrounding vascular network, however, would be of more practical benefit. The presence of ischemic or newly infarcted tissue also incorporates the rapid influx of other metabolites incorporated in the inflammatory process. These may result in diluting the concentration of isotope in a given area already deprived of available receptor sites because of a loss of viable, intact myocardial tissue. The rapid inflow and outflow of tissue fluids in an acutely infarcted area, while permitting the rapid access of nuclide to the affected area, also results in rapid washout, resulting in a decreased time for viewing the isotope in situ. Finally, while a given molecule of free fatty acid if even partially metabolized, would usually yield many two-carbon fragments and a great deal of high-energy phosphates, only one end molecule is tagged in any radionuclide preparation. Therefore, free fatty acids are very little better than glucose in providing a suitable preparation for aerobic tagging. On the other hand, uptake of a tagged glucose or polysaccharide preparation, stimulated by the infusion of insulin and potassium ion, will provide an ideal substrate and labeling agent. It is theoretically possible that free fatty acids would be more suitable for relatively normal hearts functioning aerobically, while glucose-tagged preparations would be better for ischemic areas. The theoretical advantage here, however, is negated by the fact that the extreme vascularity of the heart and rather rapid production of new collateral channels rarely leave a large area totally ischemic for any prolonged length of time.

Summary

Tailoring the isotope to the need in myocardial imaging is a complex problem, requiring basic knowledge of cardiac anatomy, and physiology, drug biochemistry, and radionuclide chemistry and technology. The problem is compounded by the rapidly changing cardiac status during any disease process. Unless all variables are in reasonable agreement, either "hot-spot" or "cold-spot" imaging will be unsatisfactory. The answers to the current state of the art and science of myocardial imaging will undoubtedly be found in reconsideration and continued exploration of the basic principles involved.

References

1. Spain, D. M., The pathologic spectrum of myocardial infarction, in: *Atherosclerosis and Coronary Heart Disease,* (J. H. Moyer, ed.) Grune & Stratton, New York (1972).
2. Roberts, W. C., Coronary artery pathology in fatal ischemic heart disease, in: *The Myocardium: Failure and Infarction* (E. Braunwald, ed.), H. P. Publishing Co., New York (1974).
3. Montgomery, G.., *Textbook of Pathology,* Vol. 1, Williams and Wilkins, Baltimore (1965).
4. Roberts, W. C., Coronary arteries in fatal acute myocardial infarction, *Circulation 45:*215 (1972).
5. Wiggers, C. J., *The Pressure Pulses in the Cardiovascular System,* Longmans, Green and Co., London (1928)
6. Sonnenblick, E. H., Correlation of myocardial ultrastructure and function, *Circulation 38:*29 (1968).
7. Schlant, R. C., Metabolism of the heart, in: *The Heart* (J. W. Hurst and R. B. Logue, eds.), Chap. 9, McGraw-Hill Book Co., New York (1970).

Potassium-43 and Rubidium-81 Myocardial Imaging at Rest, at Exercise, and During Angina Pectoris

Barry L. Zaret

Introduction

The myocardial accumulation of radioactive intracellular cations, such as potassium and rubidium, was first demonstrated by Love in 1954.[1] Eight to ten years then elapsed before Carr and his co-workers applied this observation to the study of static imaging of the myocardium.[2,3] In these prototype studies, using the model of experimental canine infarction, significant imageable radioactivity was detected within a normal left ventricular myocardium following intravenous administration of radionuclide. Regions of myocardial infarction appeared as "cold spots," or zones of relatively decreased or absent radioactivity. Following these initial studies, a number of groups have attempted to use various radionuclides to image the atherosclerotic myocardium. Most work has focused on radioactive tracers, such as potassium and ions that are capable of exchange with the myocardial intracellular cation pools. Potassium-43 was introduced as a clinical imaging radionuclide in 1971.[4] In addition to potassium, the physiologically similar monovalent cations rubidium,[5] cesium,[6] thallium,[7,8] and ammonium ion[9,10] have been employed. Other classes of compounds investigated include labeled fatty acids,[11] norepinephrine,[12] amino acids,[13] toluidine blue,[14] and bretylium analogues.[15] In all instances the region of interest, be it infarction or

BARRY L. ZARET · Departments of Internal Medicine and Diagnostic Radiology, Yale University School of Medicine, New Haven, Connecticut.

ischemic zone, is visualized as an area of decreased activity surrounded by areas of normal uptake in adjacent and/or overlying portions of the left ventricle. This undoubtedly limits resolution in comparison to that which can be obtained when the abnormal area is visualized as a "hot spot," or region of increased radioactivity, as has been demonstrated in acute infarction with the bone-imaging agents. A recent novel approach for visualizing regions of coronary stenosis or occlusion as hot spots, while employing traditional cold-spot agents, such as potassium-43, has been suggested by Cibulski *et al.*[16] This approach involves retrograde injection of tracers into the coronary sinus during transient, proximal coronary-sinus closure. The radionuclide is then maximally distributed to low-pressure–low-arterial-flow zones, and defects are seen as hot spots. Although such an approach is of interest, it obviously lacks broad clinical applicability.

Our own experience has been primarily with potassium-43 (^{43}K) and rubidium-81 (^{81}Rb) imaging in humans, and the remainder of the discussion will deal with our initial results. The goals of this approach are: (1) to visualize regions of previous myocardial infarction and hence scar; (2) to visualize zones of acute infarction, and (3) to visualize or detect regions of myocardium that are viable but transiently ischemic. The clinical implications of such an approach are clear. Such a technique can complement information obtained at the time of cardiac catheterization, help in the selection of patients for further study, hopefully serve as a screening procedure, and serve as a means of monitoring the results of therapy. In order to obtain information concerning reversible ischemia and infarction, we have combined the standard image approach with clinical exercise testing, and have studied patients both in the resting state and in association with exercise stress.

The basis for studying patients during at least two physiological states resides in the clinical observation that the occurrence of angina pectoris or transient myocardial ischemia in patients with coronary heart disease frequently requires a stress situation that alters regional myocardial supply–demand ratios. At rest, such patients are generally without symptoms. Generally, extreme reductions in arterial luminal diameter are required before blood flow and perfusion are diminished, and resting regional flow is normal or close to normal even in the presence of severe disease.

Within this context one might expect, in the absence of infarction, abnormal images or radionuclide myocardial distribution when the tracer is administered during exercise stress, in comparison with a normal resting pattern. There would be two major mechanisms for this phenomenon (Figure 1). The distribution of potassium and its analogues, rubidium and thallium, is clearly blood flow–dependent. The flow dependency of myocardial potassium and rubidium uptake has been best demonstrated in animal models by comparison of the myocardial uptake of these cations and radioactive microspheres. Under optimal experimental conditions, myocardial microsphere distribution is governed only

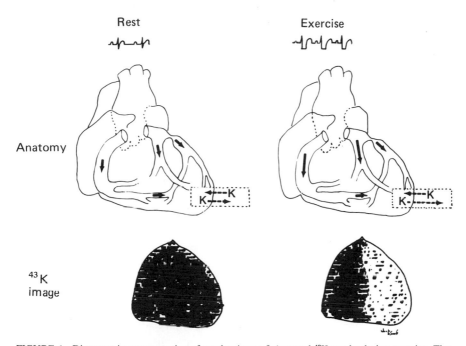

Rest

Exercise

Anatomy

^{43}K image

FIGURE 1. Diagramatic representation of mechanisms of abnormal ^{43}K uptake during exercise. The example is of single-vessel obstruction of the left anterior descending coronary artery with collateral filling from the right. The solid arrows indicate coronary blood flow, size, and magnitude of flow. During ischemia there is minimal if any increase in flow to the obstructed artery. Potassium kinetics is shown by the broken arrows. During ischemia there is altered uptake of potassium. See the text for further details. (Reproduced from Zaret et al.[22] with permission of the publisher.)

by regional blood flow. Prokop et al. demonstrated an excellent linear correlation between myocardial potassium and microsphere uptake under conditions of both infarction and graded ischemia.[17] This relationship was altered only in the condition of reactive hyperemia, during which an increase in regional potassium uptake comparable to that seen with microspheres was not present.

Under conditions of exercise stress, myocardial blood flow can increase 2- to 3-fold. The increase in flow would presumably be greatest in regions supplied by normal coronary arteries, and would be less or even absent in regions supplied by vessels with high-grade, fixed obstructions. Recent studies by Maseri suggest that during clinical angina pectoris, regional flow may even significantly decrease.[18] Thus, during exercise stress, heterogeneity in regional myocardial blood-flow responses should lead to differences in the absolute quantity of ^{43}K available for exchange in myocardial capillary beds beyond arterial obstruction in comparison to beds supplied by normal coronary arteries. Since the myocardial clearance rate and the extraction ratio of potassium are high, these relative differences in flow should be reflected in proportionate regional radioactivity concentrations in a myocardial scan or image.

During acute ischemia, metabolic factors will also govern myocardial cation uptake and balance. Intracellular cation distribution is dependent on intact cell-membrane function. This membrane function is maintained by the enzyme adenosine triphosphatase (ATPase), which helps maintain transcellular electrochemical gradients of potassium and sodium. During myocardial ischemia or hypoxia, there is a significant alteration in this membrane enzyme function, resulting in a markedly altered capability of cells to extract potassium and similar behaving intracellular cations. This phenomenon has been most recently demonstrated by Levenson et al.,[19] who utilized an animal preparation in which hypoxic blood was infused into a coronary artery under normal flow rates. Under this condition, regional radioactive cesium (^{129}Cs) uptake was definitely diminished. Another metabolic possibility would involve actual efflux of the radioactive tracer after it has been extracted. However, this latter mechanism was not demonstrated by Levenson and colleagues in the just noted model. Thus, in the circumstance of transient myocardial ischemia or angina pectoris, there are several reasons regional radioactive-cation distribution would be abnormal when administered during exercise stress, while normal under resting conditions.

In the presence of previous myocardial infarction and hence scar, the mechanisms governing potassium uptake are somewhat easier to explain. Once again, flow dependency is a factor. In the presence of infarction, extremely high-grade coronary obstructions are generally found. However, of greater significance is the presence of a markedly decreased regional intracellular cation pool, available for tracer exchange. In the case of acute infarction, this would be due to ongoing necrosis in the infarct zone; in the case of remote infarction, to replacement of normal cellular myocardium by an acellular collagen scar.

Generally, these physiologic concepts are applied to clinical procedures by studying patients on two separate occasions: at rest and during exercise stress. Studies are usually separated by approximately 2 days to allow sufficient physical decay and biological redistribution of the tracer. In the absence of infarction, it is generally best to perform the exercise study initially. If the results are unremarkable, there is no need to proceed with a resting scan. Resting studies are best performed following a 12-hr fast. Patients should receive the intravenous radionuclide in an upright posture, rather than in the supine position.

Both these maneuvers are designed to reduce hepatic and splanchnic blood flow, and hence subdiaphragmatic organ uptake of the radioactive tracer. Subdiaphragmatic activity, if excessive, can alter visualization of both the inferior wall in the anterior view and the lower septal and apical region in the left anterior oblique view. In the exercise state, during which there is a significant redistribution of splanchnic blood flow, subdiaphragmatic activity is not a problem.[20]

For exercise studies, patients undergo a graded stress test on either a treadmill or a bicycle ergometer (Figure 2). Continuous electrocardiographic monitering is employed throughout. Currently, we are using a bicycle ergometer and have this situated in the clinical nuclear medicine laboratory. The instrument takes up little room, and having the exercise capability immediately adjacent to the imaging instrument eliminates the logistic problem of patient transport in the postexercise state.

The procedure is as follows: An intravenous infusion is begun prior to exercise to facilitate tracer administration. Then the patient exercises maximally to the endpoint of severe fatigue or chest pain, at which point the radionuclide is administered. Exercise is then continued for an additional 30–45 sec to allow adequate distribution of the tracer. After this, imaging is begun. Images or scans are obtained at a time when the patient has recovered and the ECG has generally returned to the baseline. However, the radionuclide has been distributed within the myocardium during the pathophysiologic circumstance of maximal stress and/or myocardial ischemia and appears to reflect that circumstance for the hour following injection. It should be emphasized that patients must be stressed maximally and if less than maximal effort is obtained, image defects may not be seen.

Most of our imaging procedures have been performed with the 5-in. crystal rectilinear scanner. This has been necessitated by the high energy of the major gamma emissions of both ^{43}K and ^{81}Rb. These high-energy emissions result in significant collimator septal penetration and scatter, which make scintillation-

Exercise ^{43}K study

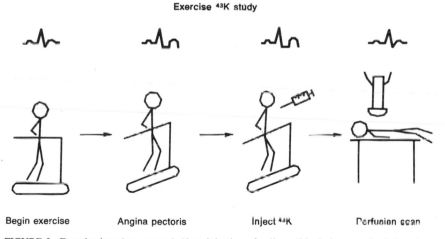

| Begin exercise | Angina pectoris | Inject ^{43}K | Perfusion scan |

FIGURE 2. Exercise-imaging protocol. Note injection of radionuclide during exercise-induced angina with imaging during the recovery period. (Reproduced from Zaret et al.[22] with permission of the publisher.)

camera imaging extremely difficult unless extensive additional lead shielding is employed in association with pin-hole collimation. This procedure is accomplished at low camera efficiency. On the other hand, with the rectilinear scanner, meaningful data can be more simply obtained without instrument modification. In this instance as well, the technique is difficult and requires meticulous attention to hot-spot calibration of the instrument for each study. We employ a 31-hole, 3-in.-depth-of-focus collimator, with the detector positioned immediately above the chest wall. Variation of the height of the collimator position can obviously alter the appearance of images by either decreasing or enhancing the perception of regional radioactivity within the optimally focused view of the crystal detector. For this reason, detector and collimator positions must be standardized from one study to another. Images are obtained with contrast enhancement (40% count-rate differential) at information densities of approximately 1000.

The high-energy spectra of both ^{43}K and ^{81}Rb point out one of the major problems with use of these radionuclides. The scintillation camera cannot be readily employed, and imaging techniques generally require more than routine technical care. These problems will, it is hoped, be overcome through the use and development of new physiologically similar radionuclides that possess more optimal physical characteristics. One such radionuclide currently under investigation is thallium-201 (^{201}Tl).[7,8] In addition, use of ^{43}K is limited by cost, cyclotron or accelerator production, and a relatively short physical half-life (22.4 hr), which necessitates frequent tracer shipment. Nevertheless, within the constraints currently imposed by radionuclide characteristics and availability, a body of clinical data has been obtained by imaging with these radionuclides.

At two institutions, over 300 patients have been studied with ^{43}K and ^{81}Rb imaging.[21-23] Rubidium-81 results have been comparable to those achieved with ^{43}K, although with the former, tracer-scintillation-camera imaging is somewhat easier. For the purposes of this discussion, data obtained with both radionuclides will be discussed together.

In normal patients, under either resting or exercise conditions, a homogeneous distribution of left ventricular ^{43}K uptake is seen. Activity is obviously present in the right ventricle and both atria, but because of their decreased cell mass, this radioactivity is not readily apparent in most scans. Frequently, a central clear space corresponding to the left ventricular cavity is appreciated. In patients with transmural infarction, studied in the resting state, regions of relatively decreased regional radioactivity have routinely been noted (Figure 3). Virtually all instances of infarction involving the anterior wall and approximately 65% of inferior wall infarcts have been detected. Difficulties in visualizing inferior wall abnormalities are due to several factors: (1) their smaller size, (2) ventricular geometry, and (3) obscuration by overlying or adjacent hepatic activity. No data are yet available in patients with subendocardial

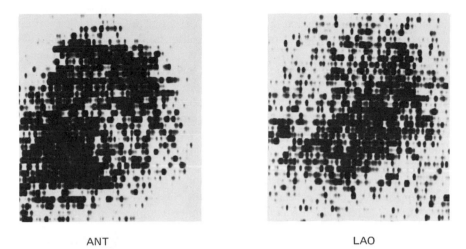

ANT   LAO

FIGURE 3. Anterior and left anterior oblique [43]K images in a patient with previous anteroseptal infarction. The region of decreased uptake is seen in both views. (Reproduced from Zaret et al.[21] with permission of the publisher.)

infarction. This experience is similar to that reported by Gorten with [43]K,[24] and Romhilt[6] and Planiol[25] with [129]Cs. Our radionuclide data have correlated well with both ECG and contrast ventriculographic estimates of the presence and site of previous myocardial infarction.

We have recently extended these observations to a semiquantitative angiographic correlative study of [43]K-defect size in patients following myocardial infarction.[26] There was a good correlation ($r = 0.77$) between the size of the defect detected by [43]K imaging and the measured extent of the ventricular circumference, which was either akinetic (without contraction) or dyskinetic (paradoxical systolic expansion). Thus, this approach appears sufficiently sensitive to allow both detection and quantitative assessment of the extent of transmural myocardial scar following infarction. In addition, in two patients, the [43]K study predicted infarction and a scar was detected at angiography that was not apparent from the surface ECG. This approach is clearly in its early stages, and a significant number of patient studies has been obtained only in patients with remote rather than acute infarction. A combination of this approach with that of hot-spot scanning of acute infarction would certainly be of interest. We have recently begun to evaluate the use of [43]K and similar types of tracers in an animal model of acute infarction with the hope of establishing the basis for quantification of infarct size with radionuclide techniques. In the case of [43]K, there is a linear relationship between the regional reduction in [43]K uptake and the extent of regional creatine phosphokinase (CPK) depletion.[27] This suggests that the cold-spot-imaging approaches may possibly be used to quantitatively assess myocardial viability in the early stages of acute infarction.

False-positive [43]K pseudoinfarct patterns have been noted in a number of clinical instances. The clinical states in which this occurs will probably increase as our experience becomes greater. These image patterns, which appear to simulate infarction, may, in fact, represent important data with respect to underlying pathophysiologic mechanisms in a variety of cardiac disease states where myocardial supply and demand relationships are adversely affected. In the case of congestive cardiomyopathy, where large ventricular cavities and decreased myocardial mass with thin ventricular walls are encountered, images simulating infarction have been regularly seen.[22] Often, in this instance, the large central defects do not extend to the outer margin of the image, and discrimination from infarction can at least be suspected. Abnormal septal uptake has been noted in patients with left bundle block and no evidence of coronary disease or cardiomyopathy. In this instance, a possible localized membrane defect involving potassium uptake has been postulated.[28] Defects in uptake have also been noted in patients with asymmetric septal hypertrophy (ASH).[29] It is of interest that in this last group, a pathologic description of intramural coronary artery abnormalities has recently been reported.[30]

The exercise-imaging technique in the evaluation of transient myocardial ischemia has been applied to over 100 patients with suspected or proved coronary heart disease, most of whom have undergone diagnostic angiographic studies. In approximately 80%, regions of relatively decreased myocardial-radioactive-cation distribution were noted on the stress study, but were either not present or present to a significantly lesser extent at rest. For the most part, these abnormalities have been noted in significantly symptomatic patients, and tracer injections have been made during chest pain, ECG changes, or both. On several occasions, initial exercise studies have been normal at subanginal heart rates, with [43]K abnormalities demonstrable only on a repeat study, during which a greater physical effort was elicited. In contrast, Berman et al.[31] have noted imaging abnormalities with [81]Rb exercise studies in a number of patients with significant coronary disease but no chest pain or ECG abnormalities during exercise testing. On the basis of these results, the authors have suggested the use of exercise-imaging procedures as screening techniques.

In our experience, abnormalities have been noted in patients with single-vessel disease of each major coronary artery as well as multivessel disease (Figures 4–6). The sites of relative decrease in [43]K or [81]Rb uptake have corresponded well to myocardial zones supplied by angiographically demonstrable stenotic coronary arteries. So-called false-positive results have been encountered in the same groups of patients in whom pseudoinfarct patterns have been noted. In these patients (with the possible exception of patients with ASH),

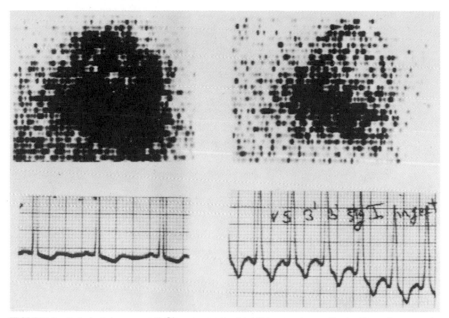

FIGURE 4. Anterior view—rest (left) and exercise (right) images in a patient with angina pectoris. ECGs at the time of injection are below each image. Note the relative decrease in uptake of the anterior wall. Arteriography demonstrated anterior descending and circumflex marginal stenosis. (Reproduced from Zaret *et al.*[21] with permission of the publisher.)

similar defects are present at both rest and exercise. False-negative results will undoubtedly present a greater problem. In patients with previous major transmural infarction, major abnormalities are usually seen in the resting scan. During exercise, additional abnormality may not be detectable, particularly if the postulated source of ischemia is in a relatively small periinfarction zone. Of greatest concern are patients with severe proximal three-vessel disease.

Imaging is dependent on demonstrating *relative differences* in myocardial distribution. In the presence of diffuse global myocardial ischemia, a homogeneous, normal-appearing study could be obtained. Although this would appear normal on a photographic scan, an expected quantitative difference in total myocardial radionuclide uptake would be expected. We have encountered this situation of false-negative exercise studies in a few patients with severe three-vessel disease or bilateral coronary ostial stenosis. In terms of single-vessel disease, false-negative results have been noted in patients with either isolated right coronary or posterior circumflex lesions.

The exercise technique has been utilized in the study of a group of patients with false-positive exercise tests.[32] This group consisted of a number of relatively young men with clinical syndromes that were not thought to represent

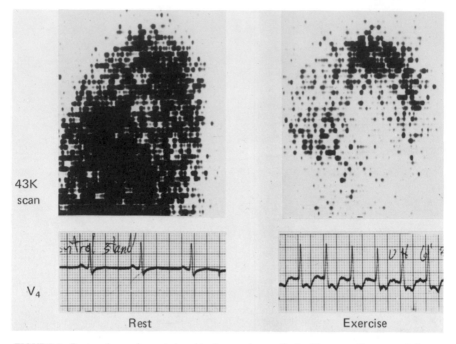

FIGURE 5. Rest and exercise anterior-view images in a patient with severe three-vessel disease. Note the marked generalized abnormality in ^{43}K uptake. The ECG during exercise shows significant ischemic changes. (Reproduced from Zaret *et al.*[21] with permission of the publisher.)

coronary artery disease, all of whom demonstrated abnormal ischemic-appearing exercise ECGs in the absence of chest pain. All patients, when studied further, demonstrated angiographically normal coronary anatomy, normal left ventricular function, and normal hemodynamics. Half the group underwent atrial pacing studies to comparable ECG changes, during which myocardial lactate metabolism was evaluated by simultaneous coronary sinus and arterial sampling. All patients so tested demonstrated normal myocardial lactate extraction, an indicator of the normal aerobic metabolic state, and therefore an indication of the absence of myocardial ischemia. All patients in this group demonstrated normal exercise ^{43}K scans, even though injection of radionuclide was made at the time of ischemic-appearing ECGs (Figure 7). Thus, the technique may be of value in screening the asymptomatic patient with an abnormal ECG during exercise.

To summarize, qualitatively demonstrable abnormalities in myocardial radioactive cation uptake have been demonstrated in patients with coronary artery disease utilizing ^{43}K and ^{81}Rb. Zones of transmural infarction can be detected at rest; zones of transient ischemia require a combination of imaging and

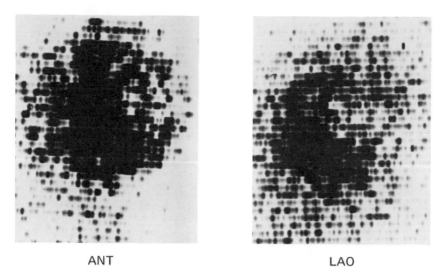

ANT   LAO

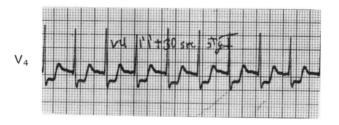

V₄

FIGURE 6. Exercise anterior- and left-anterior oblique images in a patient with right and circumflex coronary disease and posterolateral decreases in ⁴³K uptake. The ischemic ECG during exercise is below. (Reproduced from Berman et al.[32] with permission of the publisher.)

exercise stress testing. The broad clinical use of ^{43}K is limited by its physical characteristics, cost, and availability.

Future work will involve development of more optimal radionuclides for clinical use, quantification, and validation in large numbers of patients. It will be necessary to determine, in animal models, the exact physiologic and histopathologic correlates of myocardial radionuclide uptake. It will also be necessary to determine critical levels in terms of both restriction of arterial luminal diameter and restriction in flow at which defects can be detected in both resting and exercise states. Finally, it is worth looking for more rapid, simpler, possibly pharmacologic, alternatives to exercise testing for increasing myocardial blood flow and assessing coronary reserve in association with myocardial imaging procedures.

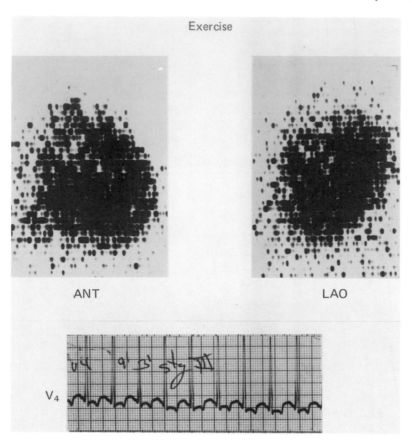

FIGURE 7. Normal exercise images in a patient with a false-positive electrocardiographic response to exercise. The ECG is below. (Reproduced from Berman *et al.*[32] with permission of the publisher.)

Acknowledgment

The author wishes to acknowledge the collaborative efforts of his colleagues M. D. Flamm, Jr., N. D. Martin, H. W. Strauss, and R. L. McGowan, David Grant, U.S.A.F. Medical Center, California; and G. S. Freedman, S. Wolfson, L. S. Cohen, R. C. Lange at Yale University School of Medicine.

References

1. Love, W. D., Romney, R. B., and Burch, G. E., A comparison of the distribution of potassium and exchangeable rubidium in the organs of the dog, using rubidium-86, *Circ. Res.* 2:112 (1954).

2. Carr, E. A., Jr., Reierwaltes, W. H., Patno, M. E., et al., The detection of experimental myocardial infarcts with photoscanning, Amer. Heart J. 64:650 (1962).

3. Carr, E. A., Jr., Gleason, F., Shaw, J., et al., The direct diagnosis of myocardial infarction by photoscanning after administration of cesium-131, Amer. Heart J. 68:627 (1964).

4. Hurley, P. J., Cooper, M., Reba, R. C., et al., ^{43}KLC: A new radiopharmaceutical for imaging the heart, J. Nucl. Med. 12:516 (1971).

5. Martin, N. D., Zaret, B. L., McGowan, R. L., et al., Rubidium-81, a new myocardial scanning agent: noninvasive regional myocardial perfusion scans at rest and exercise and comparison with potassium-43, Radiology 111:651 (1974).

6. Romhilt, D. W., Adolph, R. J., Sodd, V. J., et al., Cesium-129 myocardial scintigraphy to detect myocardial infarction, Circulation 48:1242 (1973).

7. Strauss, H. W., Lebowitz, E., and Pitt, B., Myocardial perfusion scanning with thallium-201 (abstract), Circulation 50, Suppl. III:III-26 (1974).

8. Bradley-Moore, P. K., Lebowitz, E., Greene, N. W., et al., Thallium-201 for medical use II: Biologic behavior, J. Nucl. Med. 16:156 (1975).

9. Harper, P. V., Schwartz, J., Beck, R. N. et al., Clinical myocardial imaging with nitrogen-13 ammonia, Radiology 108:613 (1973).

10. Hoop, B., Jr., Smith, T. W., Burnham, C. A., et al., Myocardial imaging with ^{13}NH$_4$+ and a multicrystal positron camera, J. Nucl. Med. 14:181 (1973).

11. Gunton, R. W., Evans, J. R., Baker, R. G., et al., Demonstration of myocardial infarction by photoscans of the heart in man, Amer. J. Cardiol. 16.482 (1965).

12. Ansari, A. N., Myocardial imaging with 11 C-norepinephrine, in: Cardiovascular Nuclear Medicine H. W. Strauss, B. Pitt, and A. E. James, Jr., eds.), C. V. Mosby, St. Louis (1974).

13. Gelbard, A. S., Clarke, J. P., and Laughlin, J. S., Enzymatic synthesis and evaluation of nitrogen-13 labelled L-asparagine for myocardial imaging, J. Nucl. Med. 15:1223 (1974).

14. Carr, E. A., Jr., Carroll, M., DiGiulio, W., et al., The use of radioiodinated toluidine blue for myocardial scintigrams, Amer. Heart J. 86:631 (1973).

15. Counsell, R. E., Yu, T., Ranode, V., et al., Radioiodinated bretyllium analogs for myocardial scanning, J. Nucl. Med. 15:991 (1974).

16. Cibulski, A. A., Markov, A., Lchan, P. H., et al., Retrograde radioisotope myocardial perfusion patterns in dogs, Circulation 50:159 (1974).

17. Prokop, E., Strauss, H. W., Shaw, J., et al., Comparison of regional myocardial perfusion determined by ionic potassium 43 to that determined by microspheres, Circulation 50:978 (1974)

18. Maseri, A., Regional myocardial blood flow in man: Evaluation of drugs, in: Cardiovascular Nuclear Medicine, H. W. Strauss, B. Pitt, and A. E. James, Jr., eds.), C. V. Mosby, St. Louis (1974).

19. Levenson, N. I., Adolph, R. J., Romhilt, D. W., et al., Effects of myocardial hypoxia and ischemia on myocardial scintigraphy, Amer. J. Cardiol. 35:251 (1975).

20. Strauss, H. W., Zaret, B. L., Martin, N. D., et al., Noninvasive evaluation of regional myocardial perfusion with potassium-43: Technique in patients with exercise induced transient myocardial ischemia, Radiology 108:85 (1973).

21. Zaret, B. L., Strauss, H. W., Martin, N. D., et al., Noninvasive regional myocardial perfusion with radioactive potassium: Study of patients at rest, exercise, and during angina pectoris, N. Engl. J. Med. 288:809 (1973).

22. Zaret, B. L., Martin, N. D., and Flamm, M. D., Jr., Myocardial imaging for the noninvasive evaluation of regional perfusion at rest and after exercise, in: Cardiovascular Nuclear Medicine (H. W. Strauss, B. Pitt, and A. E. James, Jr., eds.), C. V. Mosby, St. Louis (1974).

23. Martin, N. D., Zaret, B. L., McGowan, R. L., et al., Rubidium-81, a new myocardial scanning

agent: Noninvasive regional myocardial perfusion scans at rest and exercise and comparison with potassium-43, *Radiology 111:*651 (1974).

24. Gorten, R., Nishimura, A., and William, J. F., The diagnostic accuracy of K-43 scans in cardiac patients (abstract), *J. Nucl. Med. 15:*495 (1974).

25. Planiol, T., Brochier, M., Pellois, A., *et al.,* Dual isotope cardiac scanning in 600 cases of myocardial infarcts (abstract), *J. Nucl. Med. 15:*523 (1974).

26. Zaret, B. L., Vlay, S., Freedman, G. S., *et al.,* Quantitative correlates of resting potassium-43 perfusion following myocardial infarction in man (abstract), *Circulation 50:*Suppl III: III- 4 (1974).

27. Zaret, B. L., Donabedian, R. K., Wolfson, S., *et al.,* Dual radionuclide study of myocardial infarction: Relationships between potassium-43, technetium-99*m* pyrophosphate and myocardial creatine phosphokinase (CPK), *Clin. Res. 23,* 172A, 1975.

28. McGowan, R. L., Welch, T. G., Martin, N. D., *et al.,* Abnormal septal uptake of potassium-43 in patients with left bundle branch block and normal coronaries (abstract), *Circulation 50,* Suppl III: III-95 (1974).

29. Myers, R. W., Redwood, D. R., and Johnston, G. S., Diagnostic accuracy of stress myocardial scintigraphy (SMS) (abstract), *Circulation 50,* Suppl III: III-4 (1974).

30. McReynolds, R. A., and Roberts, W. C., Intramural coronary arteries in hypertrophic cardiomyopathy (abstract), *Amer. J. Cardiol. 35:*154 (1975).

31. Berman, D. S., Salel, A. F., DeNardo, G. L., *et al.,* Rubidium-81 imaging at rest and after exercises: Screening test for myocardial ischemia (abstract), *Circulation 50,* Suppl III:III-26 (1974).

32. Zaret, B. L., Stenson, R. E., Martin, N. D., *et al.,* Potassium-43 myocardial perfusion scanning for the noninvasive evaluation of patients with false-positive exercise tests, *Circulation 48:*1234 (1973).

Myocardial Imaging at Rest and During Stress with MAA or Microspheres

Glen W. Hamilton, James L. Ritchie, K. Lance Gould,
David R. Allen, and Milton T. English

Introduction

Myocardial imaging with isotopically tagged particles injected directly into the coronary circulation was shown to be feasible in humans by Endo *et al.*[1] Subsequent investigators demonstrated the safety and utility of this technique.[2-5]

We have studied over 250 patients following the direct coronary injection of [99m]Tc- or [113m]In-labeled macroaggregated albumin (MAA). In slightly less than half, a second isotope injection was repeated during the coronary hyperemia induced by selective injection of contrast material. This paper will discuss the methods, physiologic significance, interpretation, and clinical value of myocardial imaging at rest and during hyperemia.

Methods

Technetium-99m and Indium-113m labeled MAA was prepared specifically for intracoronary injections to contain 1.5–4.0 mCi of activity on less than 60,000 particles of MAA.[6-8] Ninety percent of the particles were from 20–40 μm in size, and none exceeded 100 μm in diameter. After completion of arteriography, a period of 2 min was allowed for coronary flow to return to basal

GLEN W. HAMILTON, JAMES L. RITCHIE, K. LANCE GOULD, DAVID R. ALLEN, and MILTON T. ENGLISH · Department of Cardiology and Nuclear Medicine, Veterans Administration Hospital, Seattle, Washington.

levels. In the resting state, [113m]In-MAA was injected into one or both coronary arteries and flushed in with 5 cc saline. The catheter position was then rechecked by a contrast injection with special attention to streaming or selective visualization of either the left anterior descending (LAD) or circumflex (CIRC) coronary arteries. After 6–10 sec following the contrast injection, ^{99m}Tc-MAA was rapidly injected into the coronary artery and flushed in with saline. The last injection coincided with the period of peak postcontrast hyperemia shown in Figure 1. The amount of contrast material used to induce coronary hyperemia was equal to the amount used for selective coronary arteriography.

Immediately following the catheterization, the patient was taken to the nuclear medicine laboratory for imaging. In the RAO, ANT, LAO, LLAT, and LPO views, 100,000–200,000 count polaroid scintiphotos were obtained for both

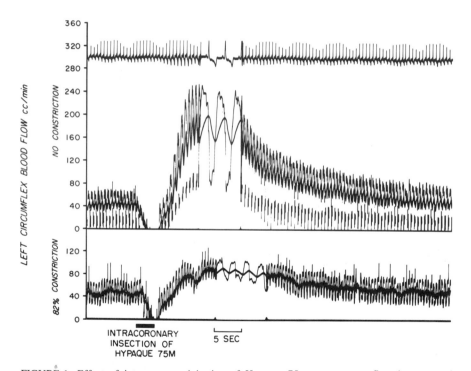

FIGURE 1. Effect of intracoronary injection of Hypaque-75m on coronary flow in a normal coronary artery and in an artery with an 82% stenosis in diameter. The flow response in the normal artery is shown above; the flow response in the artery with an 82% constriction is shown below. Resting flow in the normal and in the constricted artery are equal and approximate 40 cc/min. Following contrast injection, there is a short drop in flow and then a marked rebound increase in flow. Flow increases to 200 cc/min in the normal vessel and 80 cc/min in the constricted vessel. The flow response following intracoronary contrast material may thus be used to quantitate the degree of coronary stenosis.

isotopes and recorded directly on a computer system for analysis. Several different collimator–camera combinations were used during the study. Currently, the 400 keV converging collimator is used. Scintiphotos were interpreted by two investigators without knowledge of the clinical history or catheterization data. Computer analysis of the resting vs. the hyperemic image was performed by background subtraction and normalization of the counts in each view followed by subtraction of the hyperemic image from the resting image. This resulted in a positive image of the areas of myocardium that failed to increase flow during hyperemia.

The presence or absence of previous myocardial infarction was determined from the clinical history and ECG and was graded as none, possible, probable, or definite.[6] Coronary arteriography was performed by the Judkins technique and interpreted by at least two observers. Left ventriculography was performed, and ventricular volumes, ejection fraction (EF), and contraction pattern were determined using standard techniques.[9,10]

The Physiologic Basis for Myocardial Imaging with MAA

Small particles injected into the circulation have been shown to be distributed in proportion to regional blood flow if they are appropriately sized and injected in a manner to ensure complete mixing.[11,12] Inadequate mixing can be a significant problem with selective coronary injections. In about 5–10% of cases, streaming of contrast material into one coronary artery occurs; usually this can be corrected by catheter repositioning. If the particles are adequately mixed with blood prior to the first arterial branching, the myocardial concentration of particles injected at rest accurately represents the resting regional myocardial perfusion or blood-flow distribution. If particles are injected during periods of increased or decreased coronary flow, the distribution of particles is representative of regional blood flow under those physiologic conditions.

We have used angiographic contrast material as a convenient method to increase coronary flow. Following contrast injection, flow increases to 4–5 times resting flow (Figure 1). Injection of particles during the period of contrast-induced coronary hyperemia simulates the distribution of particles that would occur during stress. If the arterial system is normal, the distribution of particles is identical at rest and during hyperemia (Figure 2). If there is a severe arterial stenosis (generally exceeding 85% constriction by diameter), regional flow is decreased at rest, and a perfusion defect will be noted on the resting study. Stenoses of greater than 40% but less than 85% do not impair resting coronary flow, but the hyperemic-flow response following contrast injection is blunted (bottom tracer, Figure 1). The effect of a stenosis on regional distribution during contrast-induced hyperemia in an animal model is shown in Figure 2. In the first, the coronary arteries were normal, and regional distribution is identical at rest

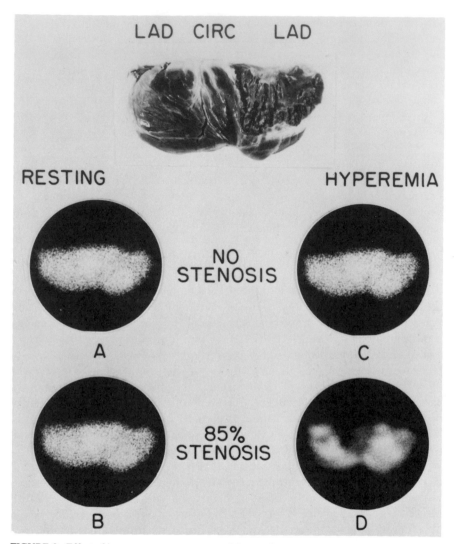

FIGURE 2. Effect of intracoronary contrast material on regional myocardial distribution in a canine heart without coronary stenosis and in a similar preparation with 85% coronary stenosis. The stenosis has been placed on the circumflex coronary artery, which is shown in the center of the top picture. Regional myocardial distribution of activity is normal in the preparation with no stenosis, both at rest and during hyperemia (A and C). In the preparation with an 85% stenosis, regional myocardial distribution is normal at rest (B); however, during contrast-induced hyperemia, relative hypoperfusion of the circumflex area occurs.

and during hyperemia (labeled as "no stenosis"). In the bottom images, an 85% constriction was induced on the circumflex coronary artery. Regional flow at rest remains normal. During hyperemia, flow increases in the LAD areas, causing a large perfusion defect in the circumflex region. The maldistribution of particles is directly related to flow abnormalities measured by an electromagnetic flowmeter ($r = 0.92$).[13,14] Additionally, both the particle maldistribution and coronary-flow response are related to the degree of coronary stenosis.[14] Thus, the distribution of particles during coronary hyperemia provides a method for assessing the physiologic significance of a particular coronary stenosis. Regional areas of myocardium with normal perfusion at rest and decreased relative perfusion during hyperemia are indicative of coronary stenosis, which limits coronary flow during periods of stress.

The Resting Myocardial Image

The pattern of the normal resting image is dependent on whether one or both coronary arteries are injected. Generally, it is most satisfactory to inject both the right and the left coronary arteries. This can be accomplished by injecting both with a single isotope ($\frac{2}{3}$ into the LCA, $\frac{1}{3}$ into the RCA), or a different isotope can be used for each coronary artery. Unfortunately, injection of both coronary arteries with one or two isotopes makes subsequent imaging during hyperemia difficult or impossible (the limitations follow). Additionally, if only the LCA is injected at rest, it is imperative to know the results of the arteriogram before interpreting the images—an apparent perfusion defect may be supplied by collateral from the other coronary artery. The term *myocardial perfusion defect* is thus limited to cases where both arteries were injected or where the area in question was shown not to be supplied by significant collaterals from the other coronary artery.

Figure 3 shows the normal regions of myocardial distribution in the LAO view. In this view, the anterior myocardium is supplied by the LAD; the posterior, by the circumflex; and the inferior, by the RCA—posterior descending coronary arteries. Figure 4 illustrates three normal myocardial images following injection of the RCA, LCA, or both coronary arteries.

Three typical abnormal images are shown in Figure 5 in the LAO view. Perfusion defects in the LAD or circumflex distribution appear as areas of diminished radioactivity. Defects in the RCA distribution (center image, Figure 5) are often accompanied by increased activity in the right ventricular myocardium if the coronary lesion is distal to the right ventricular branches.

Based on our initial 77 cases, the following relationships were noted between the myocardial image and the clinical history, ECG, coronary angiography, left ventricular angiography, surgical, and autopsy findings: Over-

Glen W. Hamilton *et al.*

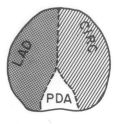

LAO VIEW

FIGURE 3. Diagrammatic representation of the coronary circulation in the LAO view. The LAD forms an anterior wedge, the circumflex forms a posterior wedge, and the PDA forms a small inferior wedge.

TABLE 1

Myocardial image	Myocardial infarction				ECG Q wave	Ejection fraction
	None	Poss.	Prob.	Def.		
Normal (36)	70%	20%	7%	3%	3%	0.63 ± 11
Abnormal (41)	2%	26%	14%	57%	66%	0.43 ± 16

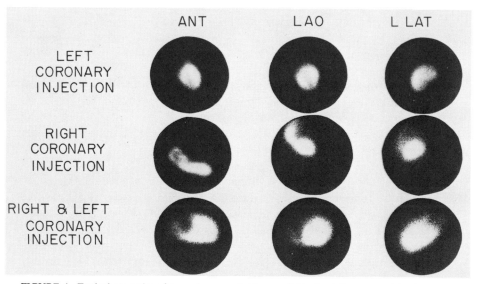

FIGURE 4. Typical examples of normal myocardial images following left coronary injection, right coronary injection, and both right and left coronary injection.

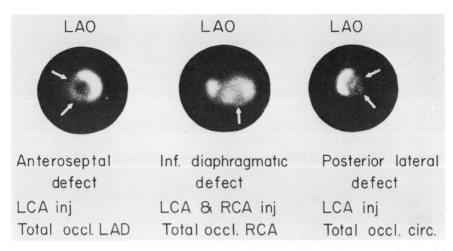

FIGURE 5. Three typical examples of resting myocardial perfusion defects due to myocardial infarction. The arrows depict the areas of the regional perfusion defect.

all, 41 patients had localized perfusion defects and 36 demonstrated normal uniform myocardial perfusion. The majority of both groups (40/41, 34/36) had angina pectoris. The presence of myocardial infarction, ECG findings, and ejection fraction is shown in Table 1 for both groups.

Of the 25 patients with definite prior myocardial infarction (ECG, Q wave, and positive history), 24 had abnormal images. Likewise, all but one of 28 patients with an ECG Q wave had an abnormal image. Localized contraction abnormalities were also more common in patients with abnormal images (58%) than in patients with normal images (7%).

No patient with coronary stenosis of less than 50% demonstrated a perfusion defect; 2 of 9 patients with stenosis of 51–75%, and 10 of 16 patients with stenosis of 75–99% had perfusion defects, 33 patients had total coronary occlusion, 29 demonstrated abnormal images, and 4 showed normal myocardial images.

In 25 cases, direct inspection of the myocardium was possible (2 autopsy, 23 surgery). In the 8 cases with normal images, none was noted to have evidence of infarction. Of the 17 cases with perfusion defects, 14 had visible scarring due to infarction in the areas of the defect, and this was confirmed histologically in 4.

In our series of resting studies, 6 of 77 patients had the syndrome of preinfarction angina. Of these, 3 had perfusion defects that could not be related to previous infarction by any of the other criteria examined. If these three are eliminated, 37 of the remaining 38 patients with abnormal images had clear evidence of prior myocardial infarction by history, ECG, contraction pattern, and/or direct inspection.

Based on these data, the following conclusions can be drawn regarding the resting myocardial image:

1. The presence of a regional perfusion defect is indicative of localized myocardial scarring due to previous infarction in the patient with chronic angina. Perfusion defects in patients with preinfarction angina may be due to scarring or infarction, but this has not been proved.
2. Myocardial imaging is a more sensitive test for the presence of infarction than the clinical history, ECG, ventriculogram, or coronary arteriogram.

Myocardial Imaging at Rest and During Contrast-Induced Coronary Hyperemia

Illustrative myocardial images at rest and during contrast-induced hyperemia are presented in Figures 6–9. In Figure 6, the resting and hyperemic images are identical, indicating the absence of previous infarction (resting image) and a normal hyperemic-flow response throughout the myocardium. Figure 7 shows a patient with a resting defect due to previous infarction that does not change during hyperemia. The patients in Figures 8 and 9 have coronary stenosis with normal resting images. During hyperemia, regional perfusion defects are

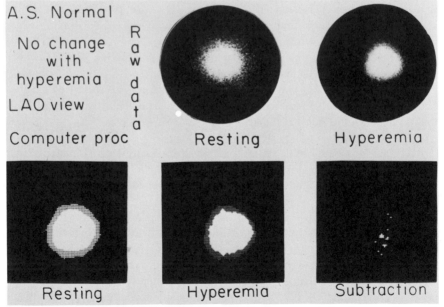

FIGURE 6. Myocardial perfusion studies at rest and following contrast-induced coronary hyperemia in a patient with no coronary disease. In the upper right, the original scintiphotos from the gamma camera are demonstrated. The lower series of scintiphotos demonstrate computer-processed images. The image during hyperemia has been subtracted from the image made at rest, and the remaining counts are presented in the lower right-hand figure. No significant change in the distribution pattern occurred.

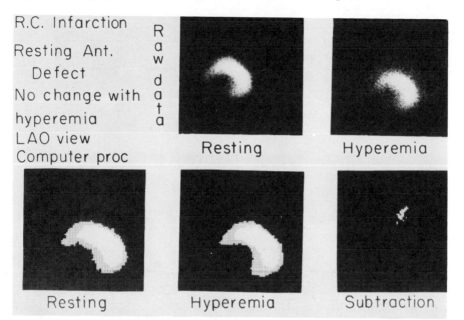

R.C. Infarction

Resting Ant. Defect

No change with hyperemia

LAO view

Computer proc

R a w   d a t a

Resting

Hyperemia

Resting

Hyperemia

Subtraction

FIGURE 7. Myocardial images at rest and during hyperemia in a patient with a large anterior myocardial infarction. The anterior defect is well visualized on the initial scintiphotos from the gamma camera and on the computer-processed images. Subtraction shows no significant change in distribution during hyperemia.

clearly seen, demonstrating that the stenoses impair regional flow during periods of increased coronary flow.

The overall results of our initial 49 studies are shown in Figure 10. The studies have been divided into four groups for analysis; normal images at rest and during hyperemia (12); normal images at rest and abnormal during hyperemia (14); abnormal images at rest, which further change during hyperemia (7); and abnormal images at rest with increased perfusion deficit during hyperemia (16). None of the patients in group (1) had previous infarction, and the coronary arteriogram was normal in 10 of the 12. All patients with normal resting images who developed perfusion defects during hyperemia had coronary stenosis exceeding 50%. In 2 of these cases, the lesion was initially missed on the arteriogram until attention was directed specifically to the artery supplying the area of the perfusion defect. Significant coronary disease was present in all patients with resting perfusion deficits.

Overall, in all 10 patients with no, or insignificant, coronary disease (< 50% stenosis), the myocardial images were normal at rest and during hyperemia. Of the 39 patients with significant coronary stenosis (> 50%), 37 demonstrated perfusion abnormalities, 14 of which were seen only during contrast-induced hyperemia.

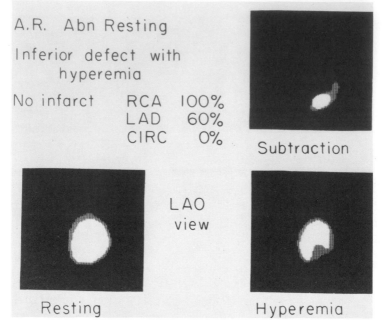

A.R. Abn Resting

Inferior defect with
      hyperemia

No infarct   RCA 100%
               LAD   60%
               CIRC   0%   Subtraction

                    LAO
                    view

    Resting   Hyperemia

FIGURE 8. Myocardial images at rest and during hyperemia in a patient with total right coronary occlusion. At rest, the myocardial image is normal. During hyperemia, a prominent inferior defect develops. The subtraction image demonstrates the precise area of the perfusion deficit.

The data from this study demonstrate that perfusion defects detected during hyperemia are indicative of physiologically significant coronary stenosis. The absence of a perfusion deficit does not, however, prove the absence of significant coronary stenosis. Equal stenosis (balanced lesions) in both the LAD and the circumflex arteries will impair flow in both, and regional perfusion defects will not be seen.[14] Additionally, the technique is most suitable for studies of the left coronary system.

In summary, myocardial imaging with ^{99m}Tc- and ^{113m}In-MAA at rest and during stress is a promising method for more accurately localizing areas of previous myocardial infarction and assessing the physiologic significance of coronary stenosis. However, certain limitations and cautions should be noted:

1. The data relating resting perfusion defects to areas of previous infarction are strong but circumstantial. These data would be strengthened by additional studies employing myocardial biopsies of normally and abnormally perfused areas during surgery.

2. The sensitivity of both techniques (i.e., detection of previous infarction and detection of significant coronary stenosis) appears favorable compared to other currently available techniques. However, the other techniques clearly have limitations in themselves.

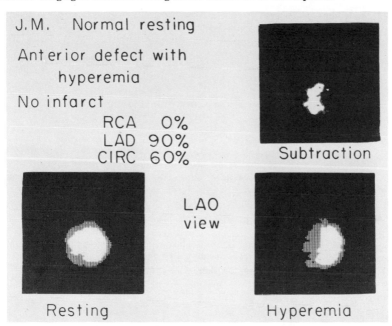

J.M. Normal resting

Anterior defect with
hyperemia

No infarct

RCA 0%
LAD 90%
CIRC 60%

Subtraction

LAO
view

Resting

Hyperemia

FIGURE 9. Typical studies at rest and during coronary hyperemia in a patient with disease in both the circumflex and left anterior descending coronary arteries. The left anterior descending artery is more severely compromised than the circumflex artery. At rest, myocardial distribution is normal. During contrast-induced hyperemia, the entire anterior half of the myocardium, normally supplied by the left anterior descending artery, shows diminished activity.

NUMBER		12	14	7	16
RESTING		NORM	NORM	ABN	ABN
HYPEREMIA		NORM	ABN	NO CHANGE	CHANGE
PERCENT WITH					
INFARCTION	NONE, POSS	100	79	14	19
	PROB, DEF	0	21	86	81
ECG Q WAVE		0	14	72	50
CONTRACTION	I, II, III,	100	93	28	62
PATTERN	III, IV, V	0	7	72	38
CORONARY	NONE	75	0	0	0
STENOSIS	< 50%	8	0	0	0
	> 50%	17	100	100	100

FIGURE 10. Relationships of myocardial imaging at rest and following contrast hyperemia to infarction, ECG Q-wave, contraction pattern, and coronary stenoses.

3. Finally, the ability to study only the left coronary artery is a serious problem, and the required use of two isotopes in the left system precludes performing the resting study with one isotope for each coronary artery.

We anticipate that further investigative, technologic, and methodologic advances will ultimately result in the solution of these current limitations.

References

1. Endo, M., Yamazaki, T., Konno, S., Hiratsuka, H., *et al.*, The direct diagnosis of human myocardial ischemia using ^{131}I-MAA via the selective coronary catheter, *Amer. Heart J. 80:*498 (1970).
2. Weller, D. A., Adolph, R. J., Wellman, H. N., *et al.*, Myocardial perfusion scintigraphy after intracoronary injection of ^{99m}Tc-Labeled human albumin microspheres, *Circulation 46:*963 (1972).
3. Jansen, C., Judkins, M. P., Grames, G. M., Gander, M., and Adams, R., Myocardial perfusion color scintigraphy with MAA, *Radiology 109:*369 (1973).
4. Schelbert, H. R., Ashburn, W. L., Covell, J. W., *et al.*, Feasibility and hazards of the intracoronary injection of radioactive serum albumin macroaggregates for external myocardial perfusion imaging, *Invest. Radiol. 6:*379 (1971).
5. Ashburn, W. L., Braunwald, E., Simon, A. L., *et al.*, Myocardial perfusion imaging with radioactive-labeled particles injected directly into the coronary circulation of patients with coronary artery disease. *Circulation 44:*851 (1971).
6. Hamilton, G. W., Ritchie, J. L., Allen, D. R., Lapin, E., and Murray, J. A., Myocardial perfusion imaging with ^{99m}Tc or ^{113m}In macroaggregated albumin: Correlation of the perfusion image with clinical, angiographic, surgical and histologic findings, *Am. Heart J. 89:*708, 1975.
7. Ritchie, J. L., Hamilton, G. W., Gould, K. L., Allen, D. R., Kennedy, J. W., and Hammer-mesiter, K. E., Myocardial imaging with ^{113m}In and ^{99m}Tc MAA: A new procedure for the identification of stress-induced regional ischemia, *Am. J. Cardiol. 35:*380, 1975.
8. Allen, D. R., Hartnet, D. E., Nelp, W. B., and Hamilton, G. W., A rapid and reliable method of labelling SN-MAA with ^{113m}InCl$_3$, *J. Nucl. Med. 15:*821 (1974).
9. Dodge, H. T., Sandler, H., Ballew, D. W., *et al.*, The use of biplane angiocardiography for measurement of left ventricular volume in man, *Amer. Heart J. 60:*762 (1960).
10. Hamilton, G. W., Murray, J. A., and Kennedy, J. W., Quantitative angiography in ischemic heart disease: The spectrum of abnormal left ventricular function and the role of abnormally contracting segments, *Circulation 45:*1065 (1972).
11. Poe, N. D., Comparative myocardial distribution patterns after intracoronary injection of cesium and labelled particles, *Radiology 106:*341 (1973).
12. Wagner, H. N., Rhodes, B. A., Sasaki, Y., *et al.*, Studies of the circulation with radioactive microspheres, *Invest. Radiol. 4:*374 (1969).
13. Gould, K. L., Lipscomb, K., and Hamilton, G. W., A physiologic basis for assessing critical coronary stenosis: Instantaneous flow response and regional distribution during coronary hyperemia as measures of coronary flow reserve, *Am. J. Cardiol. 33:*87 (1974).
14. Gould, K. L., Hamilton, G. W., Lipscomb, K., and Kennedy, J. W., A method for assessing stress induced regional malperfusion during coronary arteriography: Experimental validation and clinical application, *Am. J. Cardiol. 34:*557 (1974).

Measurement of Myocardial Blood Flow Using ^{133}Xe

Robert W. Parkey, Frederick J. Bonte,
Ernest M. Stokely, George C. Curry, and
James T. Willerson

Introduction

In 1945, Kety and Schmidt[1] devised a method to measure cerebral blood flow using a diffusible indicator, nitrous oxide. In 1949, Kety[2] substituted ^{24}Na and described the first practical method to measure blood flow using a radionuclide tracer. In the following years, some groups[3-11] elaborated further on Kety's work and developed methods for measuring myocardial blood flow by injection of diffusible tracers into a coronary artery or into the myocardium itself. The disappearance, or "washout," of radioactivity was measured by an external radiation-detection system placed over the myocardium. Kety had shown that the rate of washout of the diffusible indicator from tissue to blood was a function of tissue blood flow.[1,2,12]

The radioactive noble gases, ^{85}Kr and ^{133}Xe, have two distinct advantages over ^{24}Na and the other cation tracers: (1) the fat-soluble noble gases are capable of diffusing much more rapidly through capillary endothelium into surrounding tissues,[13] and thus can measure far higher rates of blood flow than is possible with water-soluble cations; (2) approximately 95% of a noble gas tracer bolus

ROBERT W. PARKEY, FREDERICK J. BONTE, ERNEST M. STOKELY, GEORGE C. CURRY · Department of Radiology, and JAMES T. WILLERSON · Department of Medicine, Southwestern Medical School, The University of Texas Health Science Center, Dallas, Texas.

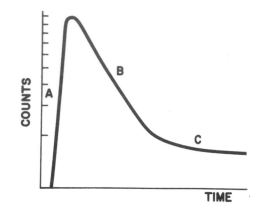

FIGURE 1. Curve recorded after intracoronary-arterial injection of a diffusible indicator such as [133]Xe. Data are plotted on a semilogarithmic scale showing counts (amount of radioactivity) as a function of time after injection. *A* designates the limb of the curve that represents the arrival of tracer in the vascular bed of interest. *B* represents blood clearance of indicator from tissue, or washout. *C*, the tail of the curve, represents washout of tracer from epicardial fat and other functions that are discussed in the text. (From Bonte *et al.*[33])

enters alveolar air at the first circulation through the lung.[14] Blood-flow washout curves (Figure 1) are thus free of secondary peaks due to recirculation of tracer. Also, one can inject successive doses of the tracer with little build-up in background radioactivity. Even though both [85]Kr and ^{133}Xe emit low-energy beta particles, the radiation dose to the patient is small because of their short biological half-life (2–4 min). [133]Xe is the present tracer of choice ([133]Xe: physical half-life = 5.27 days; γ = 80 keV; $\bar{E}\beta$ = 0.1 MeV). [127]Xe is just becoming available and could replace [133]Xe. Its longer half-life should make it less expensive to ship and store; its higher photon energy and greater abundance of usable photons provides for high resolution. The greater abundance of usable photons permits a reduction in the number of millicuries administered, while the absence of beta radiation results in reduced patient dosage [[127]Xe: physical half-life = 36.4 days; γ = 580 keV (1.4%), 145 keV (4.2%), 172 keV (22%), 203 keV (65%), 375 keV (20%); no beta].

By examining a representative procedure, one can see how blood flow is derived from a radionuclide noble gas washout curve. After a catheter has been placed in a coronary artery, a single bolus of 15–20 mCi ^{133}Xe dissolved in 1 ml normal saline is rapidly injected. A scintillation detector, such as a probe or a gamma camera, is put in place over the precordium. The radioactivity recorded by the detector is plotted as in Figure 1, with counts recorded on a logarithmic scale along the ordinate and time recorded on an ordinary scale along with the abscissa. As the bolus of ^{133}Xe appears within view of the detector, there is a sharp rise in recorded radioactivity (the *A* limb of the curve, Figure 1). When the bolus reaches the capillary bed of the myocardium, the freely diffusible xenon leaves the capillary vascular space to enter muscle, fat, and other cells that compose the heart wall. The exchanges take place in relation to

$$\frac{\text{Solubility of } ^{133}\text{Xe in myocardium muscle (or fat)}}{\text{solubility of } ^{133}\text{Xe in blood}} = \gamma$$

where the partition coefficient is γ. For ^{133}Xe in myocardium, it is usually given as 0.72, while for fat it is very high, 8.0.[13]

After the crest of the bolus passes, the blood that follows contains less tracer than the tissues surrounding capillary vessels, and the tracer begins to diffuse from the tissues back into the vascular space at a rate that is proportional to the blood flow. Note that this portion of the curve (B limb, Figure 1) described a nearly straight line on the semilogarithmic scale on which it has been plotted. It is this portion of the curve that most investigators believe represents myocardial blood flow.

Blood flow may be calculated from the washout curve by one of several methods. The original one is the Kety-Schmidt equation

$$F = (k)(\gamma)(100)/p$$

where F is the bloodflow, γ is the partition coefficient, k is the rate constant derived from the washout curve, and p is the specific gravity of myocardium. The Kety-Schmidt equation is based on a known volume of tissue perfused; inasmuch as the volume of myocardium perfused in any individual determination is not known, blood flow is expressed in terms of an arbitrary 100 g tissue, which is converted to volume by dividing by p, the specific gravity of myocardium (volume equals mass/specific gravity). The value of p is 1.05; therefore, the units in which blood flow (F) is expressed will be milliliters per minute per 100 g myocardium.

The rate constant k is the slope of the washout curve. It is derived from the semilogarithmic data plots as in Figure 6, using the equation

$$k = \frac{\log(C_1 - C_2)}{0.434\,(T_2 - T_1)}$$

where times T_1 and T_2 (see Figure 2) are selected so that the curve between them is as close as possible to a straight line. C_1 and C_2 are counts at times T_1 and T_2, respectively (Figure 2). The factor 0.434 must be used to convert the logarithm to the base 10 data so that they may be used in a log to the base e equation. It represents $\log_{10} e$.

It is evident from examination of the curve in Figure 2 that several functions

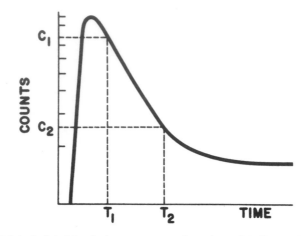

FIGURE 2. Method of deriving k, the rate constant, from the straight-line portion of the washout curve. Times T_1 and T_2 are selected so that the curve between them is as close as possible to a straight line. C_1 and C_2 are counts at times T_1 and T_2. (From Bonte *et al.*[33])

are expressed. The steep portion of the washout curve (B limb) is assumed to represent myocardial blood flow, but the origin of the long tail (C limb) has not been completely solved. It is believed to reflect, in part, washout of tracer from fat in the epicardium and body wall and clearance of ^{133}Xe from the lungs. Although 95% of the tracer bolus of ^{133}Xe leaves the blood and enters alveolar air on its first passage through the lungs, it is cleared from the lungs at a much slower rate. We have measured the ^{133}Xe pulmonary clearance half-time in dogs as 108 ± 35 sec.

It is quite likely that there are other factors, as yet unknown, that participate in the formation of the tail of the washout curve.

If the data comprising the myocardial blood-flow curve are treated by a mathematical process known as *compartmental analysis*,[15] flow "compartments" can be found corresponding to the B and C limbs (Figure 1). However, under some circumstances, the B limb itself can be resolved into two different slopes yielding two different flow rates, or compartments.[16-19] Figure 3 illustrates how some washout curves can be mathematically explained as the sum of several straight lines. This suggests multiple compartments, each with its own washout rate. Parkey *et al.*[18] monitored washout for 30 min after intracoronary injection of ^{133}Xe in dogs and extracted three compartments. The tail (C limb) was felt to represent very slow flow from fat. A shift in fractional flow from the first to the second compartment (B_1 to B_2, Figure 3) occurred after experimental coronary artery embolization. Johansson *et al.*[16] reported a monoexponential (single compartment) washout curve in dogs before arterial occlusion but there was a double exponential after occlusion. They were not considering the (C limb) tail of the curve. Horwitz *et al.*[17] found a fast and slow washout component with intramyocardial injections of ^{133}Xe in patients with coronary artery disease while monitoring for 3–5 min after injection. Flow in both components rose in most patients following the administration of nitroglycerin. Holman *et al.*[20] monitored washout of ^{133}Xe for 30 min in patients and found that three compartments were present. The fraction flow to the second compartment (B_2, Figure 3) was greater in patients with coronary artery disease.

Various explanations have been advanced for the possible existence of two compartments (B_1 and B_2, Figure 3) in the myocardial washout curve: (1) physiologically, myocardial flow may be into subepicardial and subendocardial components, which have been found to yield different flow rates with intramyocardial injection techniques.[10] (2) There could be two cell populations with different partition coefficients.[21-22] This might be argued in atherosclerotic hearts, but in the dog studies[18] this would explain the postembolus shift in flow from the first to the second compartment (B_1 to B_2, Figure 3). (3) An attractive explanation at present is primary and collateral flow.[16-19]

Further observations on this matter have been made by Stokely *et al.*,[23] who have observed dual-compartment myocardial washout curves in dogs both before and after embolization. These curves were, however, derived from relatively large myocardial regions. Stokely *et al.* have reprocessed the same data, successively reducing the size of the regions in question. As regions became smaller, the tendency toward multicompartmentation disappeared, even though counting statistics remained satisfactory. This disappeared, even though counting

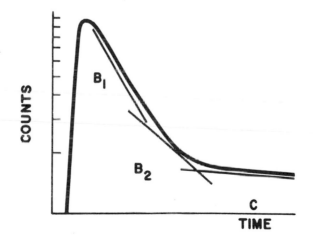

FIGURE 3. Mathematical treatment of some myocardial blood-flow curves suggests two different flow rates, or "compartments," in the myocardial washout (B, Figure 1) portion of the curve. These are represented by tangents drawn parallel to appropriate segments of the curve and identified as B_1 and B_2. (From Bonte *et al.*[33])

statistics remained satisfactory. This finding suggests that the tendency to form several flow compartments may in some way be related to the geometric distribution of both vessels and myocardium in the region being studied.

Mean Myocardial Blood Flow

If a bolus of a diffusible indicator, such as ^{133}Xe, is injected through a catheter into a coronary artery, a disappearance curve can be recorded with a single scintillation probe placed over the precordium. Flow measurements calculated from curves of this sort have been termed *total* or *mean myocardial blood flow*. Total or mean flow curves can also be obtained with the scintillation camera if the area of interest is considered to be the entire heart. The results of mean flow determination have been limited, since they often yield overlapping flow values and thus fail to distinguish between patients with radiographically demonstrable coronary artery disease and individuals with radiographically normal coronary vessels. The best explanation seems to be that coronary artery disease in relatively small areas of myocardium may cause severe symptoms and disability even though flow is normal throughout the remainder of the myocardium. However, since most of the indicator washout is occurring in the undamaged areas, mean myocardial flow may still be within the normal range.

The main advantage of a single-probe technique (measurement of mean flow) is that it is relatively inexpensive and can be performed in a standard cardiac catheterization laboratory. Horwitz *et al.*[24] utilized a mean flow technique to study patients during selective coronary angiograms. Mean myocardial flows were calculated before and after isoproterenol infusion. In patients with normal coronary vessels and in patients with angiographically defined coronary lesions, mean myocardial blood flow increased after isoproterenol. When the change in mean flow was compared with the change in cardiac output, it was apparent that in individuals wih obstructive coronary artery disease, the increment in coronary flow was low compared with the increment in total cardiac output. Most patients with coronary artery disease were unable to respond to isoproterenol stress with an appropriate increase in mean flow, and therefore the ability to distinguish between normal and abnormal coronary vasculatures using mean flow was greatly enhanced.

Regional Myocardial Blood Flow

Since mean myocardial blood flow is not always a useful index, investigators have attempted to devise methods that would reflect regional changes in the flow patterns of hearts with impaired vasculature. Early workers applied Kety's technique,[2] employing intramyocardial injection of radiosodium. This agent was ultimately replaced, first with ^{85}Kr and later with ^{133}Xe. Using intramyocardial tracer injection, Sullivan et al.[9] found a relatively uniform flow in various sites about the myocardium of normal human subjects but noted convincing inhomogeneity of flow in individuals with disease that had been demonstrated by cinecoronary arteriography. Intramyocardial injection, which was also used by other investigators,[10,17] obviously requires thoracotomy and, therefore, cannot be used in the general workup of patients thought to have coronary artery disease.

The development of scintillation cameras and computer-image data processing suggested a new instrumentational approach to several groups.[18,20,23,27-31] Two principal systems have evolved: that which the authors employ[18,23,27,28] features a large crystal scintillation camera (Nuclear-Chicago Pho/Gamma) and a dedicated PDP 8/I computer with both tape and disk-storage capabilities. Holman et al.[20] employ a similar system, only using a different type of computer storage. The authors' data are stored by the computer in a 64 × 64 matrix (the counts are not sufficiently numerous to support a finer matrix) and recorded in the form of consecutive images (or frames) of arbitrary time duration. In most studies performed with this system, a frame length of 3.6 sec has been used and the washout curve has been recorded for a total of 300 sec. However, Stokely et al.[23] have shown that 10-sec frames will provide sufficient curve detail, and a total recording time of 90 sec after the curve peak will convey sufficient information concerning the B limb to permit flow calculation with 90% accuracy.

After the passage of the bolus has been recorded, the computer is asked to display the content of several frames on the oscilloscope and areas of interest are selected, within which regional myocardial flow curves are to be generated by the computer (Figure 4). The flow value can be displayed as histograms, as in Figure 1, or as numerical values in milliliters per minute per 100 g.

The second principal instrument system for deriving regional myocardial blood flow is that of Cannon et al.[29-31] They have selected as their detector a multicrystal camera, the Bender Camera (Baird-Atomic Autofluoroscope), and have, in effect, isolated each of the 294 crystals into separate recording entities with the aid of an IBM 360/91 computer. Cannon et al.[30] have carried out their studies largely in humans; they recorded for only 39 sec following the peak of the curve, since they wish to use only that portion of the washout curve that is apt to form a straight line in a semilogarithmic plot (B limb, Figure 1) and that does not contain the tail of the curve. Flow studies are performed as an adjunct to coronary arteriography, and coronary arteriograms are used to select those crystals from which flow values are to be evoked. These investigators have noted that there is a degree of inhomogeneity in the myocardial flow values obtained in normal individuals that is greater than that observed by investigators who used intramyocardial-tracer injection to study regional flow. They have also observed that flow rates for the left ventricular myocardium exceeded those of the right ventricle and the right atrium.

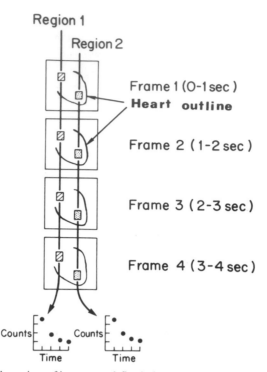

FIGURE 4. After the regions of interest are defined, the computer extracts the number of counts in each region with respect to time. The flow values can then be displayed as histograms or as numerical values.

Cannon *et al.*[31] have used this technique to appraise the success of reparative surgery with good results. Dwyer *et al.*[32] used this technique to measure perfusion in patients with residual transmural infarction. They showed that the perfusion rates observed in areas demonstrating electrocardiographic evidence of transmural infarction and regional ventricular asynergy, although subnormal, were surprisingly high and suggested the presence of residual viable myocardial cells.

Because regional myocardial blood flow has a definite advantage over only mean or total flow, this technique may find wide clinical application in the future.

References

1. Kety, S. S., and Schmidt, C. F., The determination of cerebral blood flow in man by use of nitrous oxide in low concentrations, *Amer. J. Physiol. 143:*53 (1945).
2. Kety, S. S., Measurement of regional circulation by the local clearance of radioactive sodium, *Amer. Heart J. 38:*321 (1949).

3. Cullen, M. L., and Reese, H. L., Myocardial circulatory changes measured by the clearance of NA24-effect of common duct distension of myocardial circulation, *J. Appl. Physiol.* 5:281 (1952).
4. Rees, J. R., Redding, V. J., Ashfield, R., Gibson, D., and Gavey, C. J., Myocardial blood flow measurement with ^{133}xenon-effect of glyceryl trinitrate in dogs, *Brit. Heart J.* 28:374–381 (1966).
5. Herd, J. A., Hollenberg, M., Thornburn, G. D., Kopald, H. H., and Barger, A. C., Myocardial blood flow determined with krypton-85 in unanesthetized dogs, *Amer. J. Physiol.* 203:122 (1962).
6. Ross, R. S., Ueda, K., Lichtlen, P. R., and Rees, J. R., Measurement of myocardial blood flow in animals and man by selective injection of radioactive inert gas into the coronary arteries, *Circ. Res.* 15:28 (1964).
7. Cohen, L. S., Elliott, W. C., and Gorlin, R., Measurement of myocardial blood flow using krypton-85, *Amer. J. Physiol.* 206:997 (1964).
8. Wagner, H. N., Jr., Regional blood flow measurments with krypton-85 and xenon-133, in: *Dynamic Clinical Studies with Radioisotope* (R. M. Knisely and W. W. Tauze, Eds.), Atomic Energy Commission, Oak Ridge (1964).
9. Sullivan, J. M., Taylor, W. J., Elliott, W. C., and Gorlin, R., Regional myocardial blood flow, *J. Clin. Invest.* 46:1402 (1967).
10. Brandi, G., Fam, W. M., and McGregor, M., Measurement of coronary flow in local areas of myocardium using xenon-133, *J. Appl. Physiol.* 24:446 (1968).
11. Rees, J. R., and Redding, V. J., Experimental myocardial infarction in the dog; comparison of myocardial blood flow within, near and distant from the infarct, *Circ. res.* 25:161 (1969).
12. Eckenhoff, J. E., Hafkenschiel, J. H., Harmel, M. H., Goodale, W. T., Lubin, M., Bing, R. J., and Kety, S. S., Measurement of coronary blood by the nitrous oxide method, *Amer. J. Physiol.* 152:356 (1948).
13. Conn, H. L., Jr., Equilibrium distribution of radioxenon in tissue: xenon-hemoglobin association curve, *J. Appl. Physiol.* 16:1065 (1961).
14. Holmberg, S., Luepker, R., and Varnauskas, E., Influence of recirculation on myocardial clearance curves with xenon-133, *Acta Med. Scand.* 189:241 (1971).
15. Hoedt-Rasmussen, K., Sveinsdottir, E., and Lassen, N. E., Regional cerebral blood flow in man determined by intra-arterial injection of radioactive inert gas, *Circ. Res.* 18:237 (1966).
16. Johansson, B., Linder, E., Seeman, T., Collateral blood flow in the myocardium of dogs measured with krypton-85, *Acta Physiol. Scand* 62:263 (1964).
17. Horwitz, L. D., Gorlin, R., Taylor, W. J., and Kemp, H. G., Effects of nitroglycerin on regional myocardial blood flow in coronary artery disease, *J. Clin. Invest.* 50:1578 (1971).
18. Parkey, R. W., Lewis, S. E., Stokely, E. M., and Bonte, F. J., Compartmental analysis of the ^{133}Xe regional myocardial blood-flow curve, *Radiology* 104:425 (1972).
19. Smith, S. C., Jr., Gorlin, R., Herman, M. V., Taylor, W. J., and Collins, J. J., Jr., Myocardial blood flow in man: Effects of coronary collateral circulation and coronary artery bypass surgery, *J. Clin. Invest.* 51:2556 (1972).
20. Holman, B. L., Adams, D. F., Jewitt, D., Per Eld, H., Iodine, J., Cohn, P. F., Gorlin, R., and Adelstein, S. J., Measuring regional myocardial blood flow with ^{133}Xe and the Anger camera, *Radiology* 112:99 (1974).
21. Hills, D. A., An assessment of the expression of $C = Q$ (1-exp (-$PSIQ$) for estimating capillary permeabilities, *Phys. Med. Biol.* 15:705 (1970).
22. Gosselin, R. E., and Stibitz, G. R., Rates of solute absorption from tissue depots: theoretical considerations, *Pfluegers Arch.* 318:85 (1970).
23. Stokely, E. M., Nardizzi, L. R., Parkey, R. W., and Bonte, F. J., Regional myocardial perfusion data with spatial and temporal quantization, *J. Nucl. Med.* 14:669 (1973).

24. Horwitz, L. D., Curry, G. C., Parkey, R. W., and Bonte, F. J. Differentiation of physiologically significant coronary artery lesions by coronary blood flow measurements during isoproterenol infusion, *Circulation 49:*55 (1974).
25. Conti, C. R., Pitt, B., Gundel, W. D., Friesinger, G. C., and Ross, R. S., Myocardial blood flow in pacing-induced angina, *Circulation 42:*815 (1970).
26. Klocke, F. J., and Wittenberg, S. M., Heterogeneity of coronary blood flow in human coronary artery disease and experimental myocardial infarction, *Amer. J. Cardiol. 24:*782 (1969).
27. Christensen, E. E., and Bonte, F. J., Radionuclide coronary angiography and myocardial blood flow, *Radiology 95:*497 (1970).
28. Bonte, F. J., and Christensen, E. E., Regional myocardial blood flow after experimental myocardial embolization, *J. Nucl. Med. 11:*302 (1970).
29. Cannon, P. J., Haft, J. I., and Johnson, P. M., Visual assessment of regional myocardial perfusion utilizing radioactive xenon and scintillation photography, *Circulation 40:*277 (1969).
30. Cannon, P. J., Dell, R. B., and Dwyer, E. M., Jr., Measurement of regional myocardial perfusion in man with 133-xenon and a sciintillation camera, *J. Clin. Invest. 51:*964 (1972).
31. Cannon, P. J., Dell, R. B., and Dwyer, E. M., Jr., Regional myocardial perfusion rates in patients with coronary artery disease, *J. Clin. Invest. 51:*978 (1972).
32. Dwyer, E. M., Jr., Dell, R. B., and Cannon, P. J., Regional myocardial blood flow in patients with residual anterior and inferior transmural infarction, *Circulation 48:*924 (1973).
33. Bonte, F. J., Parkey, R. W., Stokely, E. M., Lewis, S. E., Horwitz, L. D., and Curry, G. C., Radionuclide determination of myocardial blood flow, *Semin. Nucl. Med. 3:*153 (1973).

Myocardial Perfusion Imaging with MAA Following Coronary Artery Surgery

Glen W. Hamilton, Milton T. English,
James L. Ritchie, and
David R. Allen

Introduction

The primary goal of coronary surgery is the delivery of increased blood flow to regions of myocardium previously underperfused. Postoperative evaluation of coronary bypass grafts is generally performed by selective graft arteriography, which provides anatomic detail but provides little information regarding graft flow or regional distribution. Several methods have been used to evaluate bypass flow using hydrogen and xenon-133 washout[1,2] or videodensitometry.[3] None of these techniques provides information regarding the myocardial distribution of graft flow.

Direct injection of radioactive particles into the coronary graft and the coronary vessels provides accurate information concerning the distribution of graft flow.[4] However, absolute graft flow in cubic centimeters per minute cannot currently be measured. We have studied the direct particle injection method in 65 patients at the time of postoperative catheterization in an effort to evaluate the clinical utility of this procedure.

GLEN W. HAMILTON, MILTON T. ENGLISH, JAMES L. RITCHIE, and DAVID R. ALLEN ·
Department of Cardiology and Nuclear Medicine, Veterans Administration Hospital, Seattle, Washington.

Patient Material

A total of 65 patients were studied. In 34, one or more saphenous-vein bypass grafts (SVBG) were injected (45 SVBG total); in 21 patients, the SVBG was studied with one isotope and the native circulation with another isotope; in 7, internal mammary artery grafts were injected; and in 3, an SVBG was studied at rest and during contrast-induced coronary hyperemia. No particular effort was made to select patients with specific clinical or arteriographic findings, and the postoperative catheterization was considered a routine clinical procedure to assess the results of surgery.

Methods

Technetium-99m and indium-113m labeled MAA, containing 1.5 mCi and less than 60,000 particles, was used.[5] The MAA was injected directly into the graft or coronary circulation via the coronary catheter and flushed in with saline. Coronary and graft arteriography were performed using selective techniques and were recorded on both cine and large films. Filming was continued for 12 sec after the injection to ensure visualization of late collateral flow. Following the catheterization, imaging was performed with a Nuclear-Chicago HP gamma camera, using a medium-energy converging collimator. In the RAO, Ant, LAO, and LLAT positions, 200,000 count scintiphotos were obtained of both isotopes. The last 25 cases were also recorded on a dedicated computer system. Care was taken not to move the patient between the ^{99m}Tc and ^{113m}In images in any view so that regions of distribution could be superimposed. In at least one view (LAO or LLAT), 100,000 counts of both ^{113m}In and ^{99m}Tc were recorded on the same scintiphoto to further document anatomic relationships.

Coronary and graft arteriograms were read and graded by two observers in the following manner. The volume of graft flow was visually graded as: *good:* prompt graft opacification with rapid fill of the coronary vessels; *fair:* prompt graft opacification with slow but definite visualization of the coronary system; and *poor:* poor graft visualization with little or no concentration of contrast in the coronary system. The presence or absence of collateral vessels was noted.

Initially, images of myocardial distribution were read by two observers jointly and criteria were developed for the normal distribution patterns of grafts to various coronary arteries. For example, a graft to the proximal left anterior descending (LAD) should fill the entire anterior half of the myocardial image in the LAO view; an SVBG to the diagonal branch of the LAD should fill only part of this area. Later, the cases were reread without knowledge of the arteriogram and the regions of myocardium supplied were noted. In cases where both the graft and the native circulation had been injected, the superimposition scintiphotos were inspected to determine whether the entire myocardium was uniformly perfused.

Results

Injection of particles into the graft or coronary arteries caused no unto-ward symptoms and no changes in aortic pressure or ECG were noted. Imaging usually required 1–2 min and 4–5 min/view for ^{99m}Tc and ^{113m}In, respectively, resulting in a total imaging of 40–50 min/case.

Normally functioning SVBGs to various arteries presented characteristic patterns. Figures 1–3 show SVBGs to the right coronary artery (RCA), left anterior descending (LAD), and circumflex (CIRC). The left lateral and LAO views were the most useful due to the better anatomic definition of the regions supplied by the coronary arteries. SVBGs to the RCA had a "ball and tail" configuration (LAO view, Figure 1); the tail is usually less intense and represents flow to the right ventricular myocardium, while the ball represents flow to the inferior diaphragmatic left ventricle. Grafts to the LAD and CIRC often appear

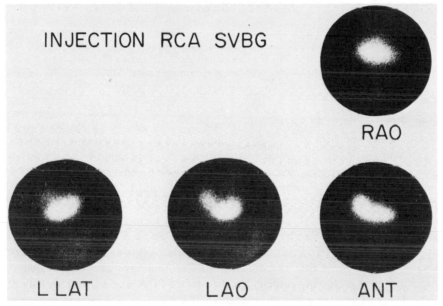

FIGURES 1. Scintiphotos of a saphenous-vein bypass graft (SVBG) to the distal right coronary artery (RCA). The "ball and tail" configuration is best appreciated in the LAO view. The tail represents flow to the right ventricular myocardium and the ball represents flow to the inferior myocardium, supplied by the posterior descending coronary artery. (LLAT) Left lateral; (LAO) left anterior oblique; (RAO) right anterior oblique.

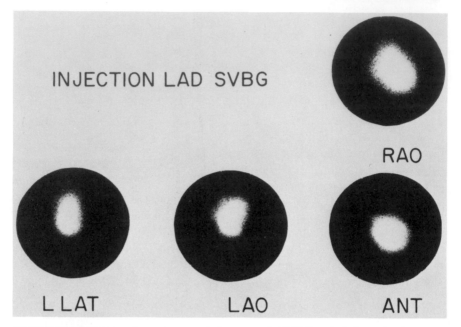

FIGURE 2. Scintiphotos of a saphenous-vein bypass graft (SVBG) to the left anterior descending coronary artery (LAD). In the anterior (ANT) and right anterior oblique (RAO), the entire left ventricle appears to be visualized. The left anterior oblique (LAO) and the left lateral (LLAT) views clearly show the activity to be anterior representing the anterior, septal, and anterolateral portion of the left ventricular myocardium.

similar in the ANT or RAO views (Figures 2 and 3). The LAO and LLAT views clearly show the activity to be anterior (LAD) or posterior (CIRC).

Comparison of the myocardial distribution following coronary artery injection (preoperatively) and graft injection (postoperatively) was possible in one patient who had separate ostia for the CIRC and LAD arteries. Figure 4 compares the myocardial distribution of a selective LAD injection to the SVBG injection; in both, the LAD area appears essentially identical. The LAD injection shows flow to the PDA area (most easily seen on the LLAT view), which is not apparent on the SVBG–LAD injection postoperatively. Injection of the CIRC and SVBG to the CIRC demonstrate similar findings. The CIRC area of myocardium is essentially similar, but flow to the PDA area is apparent only on the selective CIRC injection (best seen in RAO view). Angiography revealed collateral flow from the LAD to the PDA preoperatively but not postoperatively. Collateral flow from the CIRC to the PDA was not seen by angiography pre- or postoperatively.

Figure 5 shows single and composite views of a patient with SVBGs to both the LAD and the circumflex coronary arteries. In the LAO and the LLAT views,

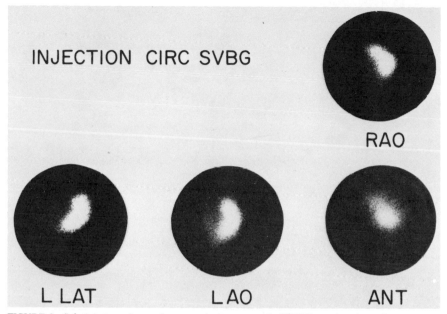

FIGURE 3. Scintiphotos of a saphenous-vein bypass graft (SVBG) to the circumflex coronary artery. The pattern of activity resembles a SVBG to the left anterior descending (LAD) in the anterior and right anterior oblique (RAO) images. On the left lateral (LLAT) and left anterior oblique (LAO) views, the area of activity is clearly seen to be posterior in the posterior and posterior-lateral part of the left ventricular myocardium. (CIRC) Circumflex coronary artery.

there is some overlap of the CIRC and the LAD areas, but they can be clearly distinguished from each other. Note also that the entire myocardium normally supplied by the left coronary artery is visualized and appears uniform. If the SVBGs are distal to the lateral ventricular branches of either artery or these branches become obstructed, a void, or region of diminished activity, between the LAD and the CIRC areas will be seen.

Collateral flow to areas other than those primarily grafted was easily visualized. Figure 6 shows an SVBG to the LAD with collateral flow to the PDA and the CIRC areas compared to a LAD SVBG without collateral flow. Collateral flow to the PDA is very intense in this case and is easily appreciated to be of greater magnitude than collateral flow to the CIRC area. In general, collateral flow to areas other than that primarily grafted was seen more frequently by myocardial perfusion studies (53%) than by angiography (18%). Additionally, the magnitude of the collateral flow could be judged by comparing the activity in the primary area to the area supplied by collateral flow.

Of the total of 76 grafts studied, 5 were judged to have abnormally small areas of myocardial distribution. All 5 showed poor flow by angiography.

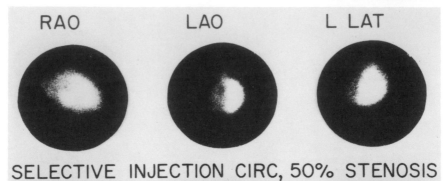

RAO   LAO   L LAT

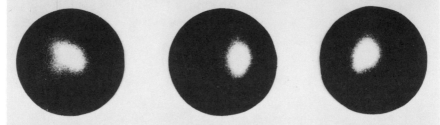

SELECTIVE INJECTION CIRC, 50% STENOSIS

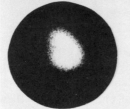 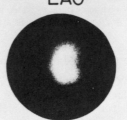 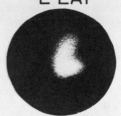

A SELECTIVE INJECTION CIRC SVBG   Pt. D.H.

RAO   LAO   L LAT

SELECTIVE INJECTION LAD, 70% STENOSIS

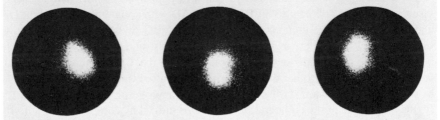

B SELECTIVE INJECTION LAD SVBG

However, 5 additional grafts with poor flow by angiography had normal-sized areas of distribution. Notable was one case with an LAD graft that showed a large area of anterior myocardial distribution, judged to be normal by MAA study. SVBG flow was poor by arteriography, and a stenosis was present at the anastamotic site; subsequent flow measurement during reoperation demonstrated a flow rate of only 15 cc/min. The MAA perfusion study thus appears to be a poor indicator of the amount of graft flow. SVBGs noted to have collateral flow on the MAA study were all judged to have good flow by arteriography, and this finding may well be indicative of good graft function.

Illustrative examples of the 7 cases in which internal mammary-to-LAD grafts were injected are shown in Figure 7. The distribution of flow to the mediastinum was surprising. Of the 7 cases, 3 showed predominant flow to the mediastinum rather than the myocardium, 2 demonstrated flow primarily to the myocardium (right image, Figure 7), and in 2, flow was distributed to both the myocardium and the mediastinum (center image). The overall distribution of flow was more obvious on the MAA study than by arteriography. Figure 8 compares an internal mammary graft with an SVBG in the same patient. The SVBG supplies only myocardium; the internal mammary graft supplies, predominantly, mediastinum.

Injection of the SVBG with one isotope and the native circulation with a second isotope was generally more useful than SVBG injection alone. Of the 21 cases, 10 showed arteriographically complete obstruction of the grafted vessel proximal to the graft at the site of preoperative stenosis. In these, the MAA study added little information; graft flow was all distributed to the primarily grafted area and the native circulation to the remaining coronary bed. Of the remaining eleven cases in which the grafted vessel remained patent, 5 showed a myocardial distribution pattern that could not be predicted by the arteriogram. Figure 9 illustrates this phenomenon. Arteriographic injection of the left coronary artery filled both the LAD and the circumflex arteries equally well. Injection of the SVBG with contrast filled mainly the circumflex with some retrograde flow to the LCA and the LAD. The MAA study showed that, in fact, flow in the LCA was all into the

FIGURE 4. Scintiphotos of (a) a single patient with a 50% circumflex (CIRC) stenosis and (b) a 70% left anterior descending (LAD) stenosis and a total occlusion of the right coronary artery. The upper images in (a) and (b) were made by selective injection of the CIRC (a) and the LAD (b). Separate ostia for the LAD and circumflex made the selective injection possible. The lower images followed selective injection of saphenous-vein bypass grafts (SVBG) to the LAD and the CIRC, respectively. The primary LAD and CIRC areas are the same in both studies. However, collateral flow to the inferior left ventricle normally supplied by the right coronary artery was more prominent in the preoperative study than in the SVBG study. The inferior collateral flow is best visualized on the right anterior oblique (RAO) and left lateral (LLAT) images in (b) and on the RAO and left anterior oblique (LAO) in (a). Angiography demonstrated LAD to right coronary collateral on the preoperative study. No angiographic collateral was noted on the circumflex injection preoperatively or on the SVBG injections postoperatively.

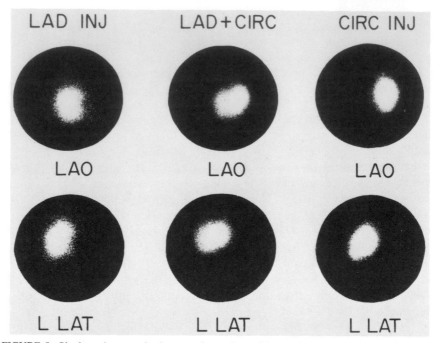

FIGURE 5. Single and composite images of a patient with saphenous-vein bypass grafts to the circumflex (CIRC) and left anterior descending (LAD) coronary arteries. The composite (LAD + CIRC) image was made by superimposing 50,000 counts of both the ^{99m}Tc window and the ^{113m}In window on the same polaroid film. The relationship of the LAD and CIRC areas is easily appreciated. (LAO) Left anterior oblique; (LLAT) left lateral.

LAD area, and SVBG flow was all to the CIRC area. Additionally, in 3 cases, areas of decreased activity were seen between the area grafted and the remaining native circulation due to failure to provide complete revascularization.

Discussion

Our interest in perfusion studies of grafts with MAA was stimulated by a difficulty in objectively evaluating the results of surgery by standard arteriography. We thought the size of the area of myocardium supplied by the SVBG might be an indicator of the volume flow in the graft. Although volume flow is difficult to evaluate by arteriography, the data presented lend little support for that concept. In fact, it appears that the size of region of myocardium supplied is a poor indicator of graft flow. The presence of collateral flow was, however, more easily appreciated on the MAA study, and the findings of collateral flow was uniformly associated with graft flow judged to be good by arteriography.

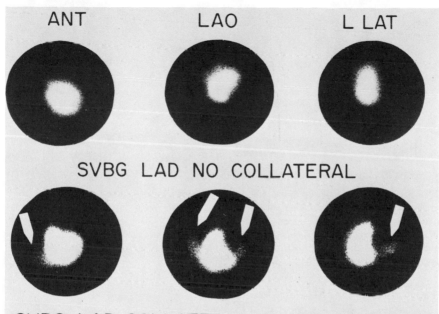

FIGURE 6. Images of two normal saphenous-vein bypass grafts (SVBG) to the anterior descending coronary artery (LAD). The upper study shows no collateral flow, while the lower images demonstrate collateral flow to both the right coronary area and the circumflex coronary area. The arrows point to areas of collateral flow. Angiographically, collateral flow was noted to the right coronary area but not to the circumflex area.

The major utility of the MAA perfusion study was the ability to more accurately assess the regional distribution of the injected arterial system. Contrast injection markedly alters coronary hemodynamics,[6-8] and it is not surprising that regional flow is more accurately ascertained by particle-injection studies. This disparity between the arteriographically predicted regional distribution and actual regional distribution measured by MAA was particularly striking in internal mammary artery grafts and in SVBGs in which the grafted vessel remained patent proximally.

Clinically, the role of this technique is uncertain. It seems likely that methods for measuring the volume of graft flow will be needed to complement distribution studies of the type used here. In the absence of graft-flow data, resting regional myocardial distribution studies are clearly of limited value. We are attempting to develop methods for measuring flow from the time-activity curve recorded during the graft injection. Until these methods are developed, routine graft-injection studies with MAA on a clinical basis does not seem warranted.

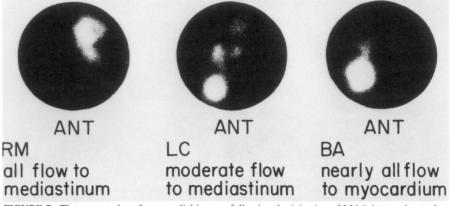

FIGURE 7. Three examples of myocardial images following the injection of MAA into an internal mammary, left anterior descending graft. In the figure on the right, most of the activity is in the anterior myocardium in the area normally supplied by the LAD. In the figure on the left, the majority of the activity is in the superior mediastinum. The center image shows the predominant activity in the anterior myocardium with a significant but lesser amount in the superior and middle mediastinal areas.

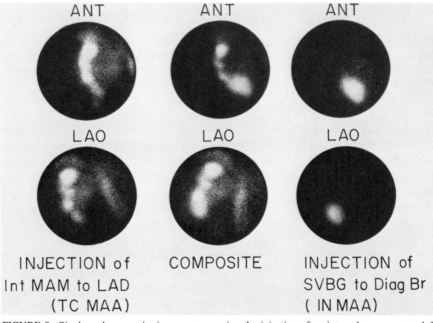

FIGURE 8. Single and composite images, comparing the injection of an internal mammary to left anterior descending graft and images following the injection of a saphenous-vein bypass graft to the diagonal branch. The saphenous vein shown on the right delivers all the activity to the anterior descending area. From the center and left images, it is appreciated that a significant portion of the activity injected via the internal mammary graft is, in fact, delivered to the mediastinum rather than to the LAD area.

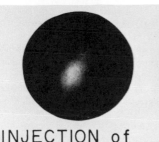 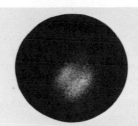 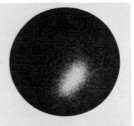

INJECTION of   COMPOSITE   INJECTION of
LCA   SVBG to CIRC

ANGIO: GOOD FLOW SVBG TO CIRC
LCA INJ FILLS BOTH LAD & CIRC

FIGURE 9. MAA images following the injection of the main left coronary artery and the injection of a saphenous-vein bypass graft to the circumflex coronary artery. The composite image was made by superimposing counts of indium and technetium activity on the same scintiphoto. The activity from the left coronary artery injection is delivered completely to the left anterior descending area while that injected via the saphenous-vein-bypass graft circumflex is delivered entirely to the circumflex area. In contrast, the coronary arteriogram demonstrated flow to both the LAD and circumflex areas when the main left coronary artery was injected.

Injection of the graft with MAA at rest and during contrast hyperemia (or other forms of stress) might prove more valuable than resting studies alone. The three cases we have performed to date are insufficient for analysis. Potentially, the distribution of flow during stress could be very different than at rest and provide additional physiologic information. A graft that supplies its primary area at rest and also supplies collateral flow to other areas during stress is likely to be of greater importance than a graft that supplies only one region of myocardium.

References

1. Greene, D. G., Klocke, F. J., Schimert, G. L. et al., Evaluation of venous bypass grafts from aorta to coronary artery by inert gas desaturation and direct flow meter techniques, J. Clin. Invest. 51:191 (1972).
2. Lichtlen, P., Moccetti, T., Halter, J., Schönbeck, M., and Senning, A., Postoperative evaluation of myocardial blood flow in Aorta-to-coronary artery vein bypass grafts using the xenon-residue detection technique, Circulation 46:445 (1972).
3. Smith, H. C., Frye, R. L., Davis, G. D., et al., Measurement of flow in saphenous vein–coronary artry grafts by roentgen videodensitometry. Circulation (Suppl. to Vol. 43) 44:389 (1971).
4. Hamilton, G. W., Murray, J. A., Lapin, E., Allen, D. R., Hammermeister, K. E., and Ritchie, J. L., Evaluation of myocardial perfusion by direct injection of radioactive particles following coronary bypass surgery, in: Coronary Artery Medicine and Surgery: Concepts and Controversies (John C. Norman, ed.), pp. 860–867, Appleton-Century-Crofts, New York (1975).

5. Allen, D. R., Harnet, D. E., Nelp, W. B., and Hamilton, G. W., A rapid and reliable method of labelling SN-MAA with $^{113m}InCl_3$, *J Nucl. Med. 15:*821 (1974).
6. Gould, K. L., Lipscomb, K., and Hamilton, G. W., A physiologic basis for assessing critical coronary stenosis: instantaneous flow response and regional distribution during coronary hyperemia as measures of coronary flow reserve, *Amer. J. Cardiol. 33:*87 (1974).
7. Gould, K. L., Hamilton, G. W., Lipscomb, K., and Kennedy, J. W., A method for assessing stress induced regional malperfusion during coronary arteriography: Experimental validation and clinical application, *Amer. J. Cardiol. 34:*557 (1974).
8. Kloster, F. E., Friesen, W. G., Green, G. S., and Judkins, M. P., Effects of coronary arteriography on myocardial blood flow, *Circulation 46:*438 (1972).

Rest and Exercise Myocardial Imaging in the Assessment of the Postoperative Cardiac Patient

Barry L. Zaret

Introduction

An obvious application of the rest-and-exercise myocardial-imaging approach would be the study of patients having undergone aortocoronary bypass surgery. The recent introduction of this surgical modality has significantly altered the therapeutic approach toward patients with coronary heart disease. Coronary revascularization procedures are now being performed in patients representing the entire spectrum of coronary disease, ranging from the situation of minimally symptomatic angina pectoris to cardiogenic shock. However, postoperative subjective improvement may not, in all cases, be due to increased myocardial perfusion. Reduction or elimination of symptoms in the individual patient may also result from perioperative infarction of ischemic muscle, partial denervation, or placebo effect. On the other hand, symptoms may persist in the presence of entirely patent bypass grafts. Dispute currently rages as to whether the procedure, even in the face of symptomatic improvement, will have a long-term effect on patient survival and prognosis. Definitive objective evaluation of the postoperative patient has required cardiac catheterization and contrast angiography, which by their very nature are limited in terms of sequential study. For this reason, a noninvasive means of evaluating graft patency and myocardial

BARRY L. ZARET · Departments of Internal Medicine and Diagnostic Radiology, Yale University School of Medicine, New Haven, Connecticut.

viability would have definite clinical and investigative value. To this end, we have applied rest and exercise ^{43}K and ^{81}Rb myocardial imaging to the study of the postoperative patient.

The technique of patient study has already been presented in Chapter 7, and will not be elaborated on further. Our initial reported series involved 16 patients in whom ^{43}K imaging was compared to cardiac catheterization and angiographic evaluation.[1] This group has since been expanded to include an additional 20 patients with comparable results. The results of imaging studies have allowed separation of postoperative patients into two distinct groups. The first group consists of patients in whom postoperative studies obtained during both rest and exercise states were normal, or patients in whom postoperative exercise studies showed either normalization or significant improvement when compared to abnormal preoperative studies (Figures 1 and 2). Patients in this group all demonstrated at least one patent bypass graft. For the group as a whole, 80% of all bypass grafts were patent at the time of angiographic evaluation. There has been good correlation between the anatomic site of coronary arterial stenosis and preoperative radionuclide abnormality as well as between demonstrable graft patency and the site of increased ^{43}K or ^{81}Rb uptake postoperatively. Clincially, all patients in this group had either diminution or absence of symptoms. It should again be emphasized that with this technique, in the absence of infarction,

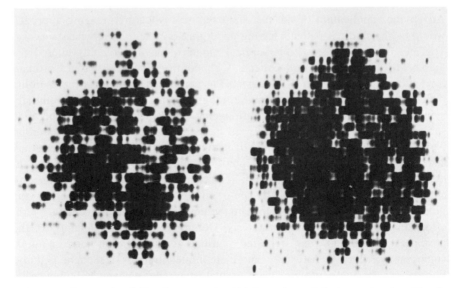

FIGURE 1. Preoperative (left) and postoperative (right) exercise study in the anterior view. Note the increase in the anterolateral wall relative ^{43}K uptake. Angiography demonstrated patent rights and circumflex grafts and an anterior descending graft with 50–70% stenosis at the distal anastamosis site. (Reproduced from Zaret et al.[1] with permission of the publisher.)

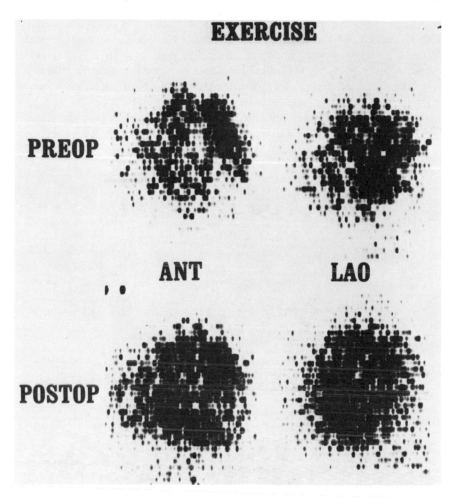

FIGURE 2. Preoperative (upper panel) and postoperative (lower panel) exercise ^{43}K images in a patient with two of three patent grafts (anterior descending and right coronary arteries). Note the significant change following surgery. (Reproduced from Zaret et al.[1] with permission of the publisher.)

preoperative abnormality and/or postoperative improvement were apparent only on images obtained with injection of ^{43}K or ^{81}Rb during exercise stress.

The second group consists of patients in whom postoperative rest and exercise studies were either not significantly different from an abnormal preoperative study or had actually worsened. When evaluated angiographically, this group is somewhat more heterogeneous. The most common situation has involved perioperative infarction, noted by imaging techniques in 6 patients. This was reflected in the occurrence of resting scan defects not present during preoperative study (Figures 3 and 4). Similar defects were noted as well during exercise study. Of the 6 patients, 4 were improved clinically, both subjectively in terms of symptoms and objectively in terms of measured exercise tolerance. In all patients with infarction, left ventriculography demonstrated significant akinetic zones, while ECGs were diagnostic in only 4 of 6 patients. Persistent postoperative exercise abnormalities have been noted in patients with patent grafts but significant new distal native obstructive coronary disease, in patients with totally oc-

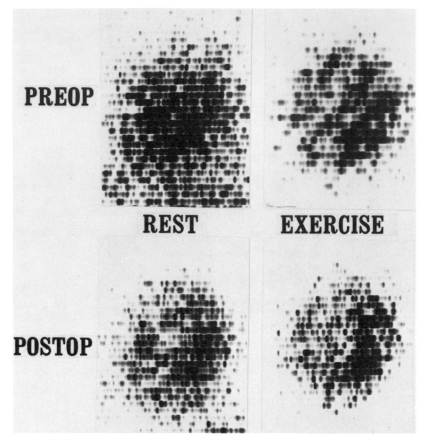

FIGURE 3. Left anterior oblique view [43]K images at rest and exercise preoperatively (upper panel) and postoperatively (lower panel). The patient had isolated involvement of the left anterior descending coronary artery. A single bypass graft was placed that subsequently occluded resulting in anteroseptal infarction. Preoperatively, note the normal resting study and abnormality associated with exercise in the anteroseptal distribution. Postoperatively, decreased anteroseptal [43]K uptake is present at rest as well, indicating interim infarction.

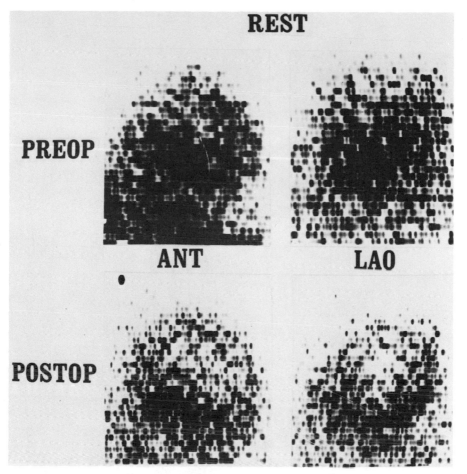

FIGURE 4. Resting ^{43}K imaging preoperatively (upper panel) and postoperatively (lower panel). Note the occurrence of a large resting anterior wall, definite in ^{40}K uptake following surgery. Postoperative infarction was confirmed by angiography. (Reproduced from Zaret et al.[1] with permission of the publisher.)

cluded grafts without infarction, and in patients with stenosis at the site of graft—coronary artery anastamosis (Figure 5). In this group as well, there has been good anatomic correlation between radionuclide and angiographic studies. Patients in these latter groups have generally not demonstrated clinical improvement.

Thus, rest-and-exercise imaging can generally furnish an objective assessment of the physiologic status of patients following revascularization surgery. With this as yet a qualitative approach, the study of patients during rest and stress is mandatory. The presence of postoperative abnormality with exercise imaging

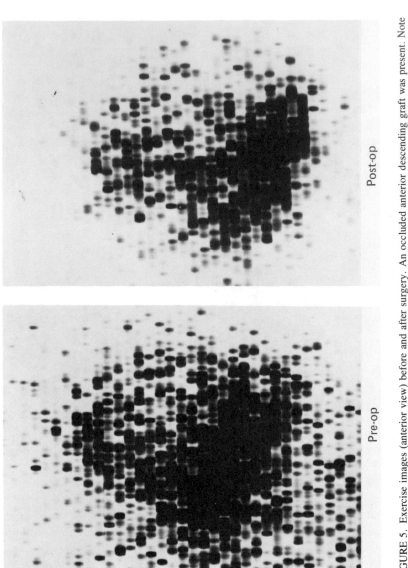

FIGURE 5. Exercise images (anterior view) before and after surgery. An occluded anterior descending graft was present. Note the absence of change in the ^{43}K image. (Modified from Zaret *et al.*[1] with permission of the publisher.)

cannot define the mechanism of apparent postoperative ischemia, but it can serve to localize the site of ineffective revascularization.

As can be surmised from the previous discussion of this technique, there are circumstances in which rest-and-exercise imaging might be expected to furnish ineffective or erroneous data. The presence of major transmural infarction prior to surgery will lead to a major preoperative and postoperative abnormality that may obscure improvement resulting from increased perfusion to a periinfarction ischemic zone. Patients with severe proximal three-vessel disease may demonstrate falsely negative normal-appearing preoperative exercise images with a homogeneous, albeit globally decreased, radioactive-cation myocardial uptake in the presence of generalized ischemia. Postoperatively, one or two of three grafts may be patent and the patient's condition may be improved. However, exercise imaging at this time may demonstrate abnormalities, since now, because of selective graft patency, a greater heterogeneity of flow and hence regional ischemia has been established, and *relative differences* in regional potassium or rubidium uptake can be detected. It is clear that a much larger group of this heterogeneous postoperative patient population must be studied before clinical efficacy can be established.

Two other approaches to the use of [43]K imaging for evaluating the results of bypass surgery have been employed; both involve study of patients in the resting state in association with computerization of data. The approach of Smith *et al.*[2] involves infusion rather than bolus injection of radionuclide, with serial acquisition of data, rectilinear scanning, and generation of functional images. This allows determination of regional appearance times and net rates of uptake.[2] Initial studies have correlated well with angiographic evaluation in a small group of patients. The technique of Botti *et al.*[3] involved three-dimension computer processing of scintillation-camera myocardial [43]K distribution.

We are presently evaluating, as well, resting [43]K imaging in a group of patients undergoing another type of surgical procedure for coronary artery disease: left-ventricular-aneurysm resection. This was undertaken to evaluate the extent of residual scar in the left ventricle following surgery. We have recently shown that in the resting state following myocardial infarction, there is a good correlation between the size of the [43]K defect and the extent of ventricular scar as assessed by measurement of segmental contraction abnormalities by quantitative angiographic techniques.[4] This same approach was applied to the postoperative patient. In all 13 patients studied following aneurysm resection, there were large residual postoperative resting defects that would be indistinguishable from the familiar pattern of transmural infarction (Figure 6). These defects averaged 40% of the image in two views. As might be expected, total image size in the anterior view decreased from the pre- to postoperative state. The extent of residual scar did not appear to affect clinical status in that, in so far as could be assessed, all

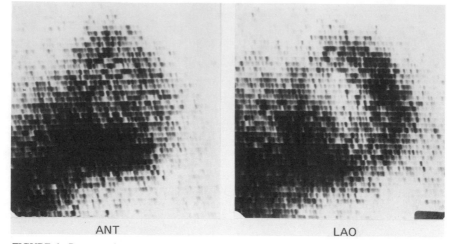

ANT   LAO

FIGURE 6. Postoperative anterior and LAO [43]K images following left-ventricular-aneurysm resection. Note the large anterior and apical abnormality that would be indistinguishable from the pattern seen in major transmural infarction.

patients had improved clinically. Although a certain degree of residual scar was expected following aneurysm resection, the magnitude of abnormality, as assessed by [43]K imaging, was greater than anticipated. This observation is currently being further evaluated in our laboratory.

To summarize, rest and exercise imaging with [43]K and [81]Rb can be used to evaluate patients following surgery for coronary artery disease in a variety of ways. These approaches obviously need technical refinement, application of quantitative techniques, and study of large numbers of patients. The approach may furnish relevant observations into the physiologic status of the postoperative coronary patient.

Acknowledgment

This study was supported by a grant from the Connecticut Heart Association.

References

1. Zaret, B. L., Martin, N. D., McGowan, R. L., et al., Rest and exercise potassium-43 myocardial perfusion imaging for the noninvasive evaluation of aortocoronary bypass surgery, Circulation 49:688 (1974).
2. Smith, R. O., Bennett, K. R., Suzuki, A., et al., Atraumatic evaluation of myocardial revascularization procedures with [43]K, Radiology 114:99 (1975).

3. Botti, R. E., and MacIntyre, W. J., Evaluation of surgical revascularization of the myocardium by peripheral ^{43}K injection (abstract), *Circulation 43:* (Suppl IV): IV-118 (1973).

4. Zaret, B. I., Vlay, S., Freedman, G. S., *et al.,* Quantitative correlates of resting potassium-43 perfusion following myocardial infarction in man (abstract), *Circulation 50,* (Suppl III): III-4 (1974).

Acute Myocardial Infarct Imaging with ^{99m}Tc Stannous Pyrophosphate

Robert W. Parkey, Frederick J. Bonte,

Ernest M. Stokely, L. Maximilian Buja, and

James T. Willerson

Introduction

A number of radiopharmaceuticals have been shown to concentrate in acutely infarcted myocardium. These include ^{203}Hg-chlormerodrin,[1,2] ^{203}Hg-mercurifluorescein,[3,4] ^{99m}Tc-tetracycline,[5] ^{67}Ga,[6] ^{99m}Tc-glucohepatonate,[7] and ^{99m}Tc-phosphates.[7,8] The best images to date have been with ^{99}Tc-stannous pyrophosphate (^{99m}Tc-PYP).[9-11]

Why do the ^{99m}Tc-phosphates localize in acutely infarcted myocardium? The final answer is not known at this time, but it continues to appear that the ^{99m}Tc-PYP localizes in a calcium phosphate crystalline structure. D'Agostino and Chiga[12,13] described the localization of calcium ions within the mitochondria of necrotic myocardial cells and observed that the calcium seemed to be incorporated in hydroxyapatite. Shew and Jennings[14,15] gave ^{45}CaCl$_2$ to dogs after occlusion of the coronary artery for varying time intervals and drew two conclusions: (1) calcium uptake is a feature of irreversible cellular injury only when arterial blood flow is present, and (2) calcium uptake behaves as if it were

ROBERT W. PARKEY, FREDERICK J. BONTE, and ERNEST M. STOKELY · Department of Radiology, L. MAXIMILIAN BUJA · Department of Pathology, and JAMES T. WILLERSON · Department of Medicine, Southwestern Medical School, The University of Texas Health Science Center, Dallas, Texas.

an active process associated with mitochondrial accumulation of calcium in granules of calcium phosphate. Our studies[16] show that ^{99m}Tc-PYP is located in the infarct, where the maximum calcification is present, although the amounts of ^{99m}Tc-PYP and Ca do not always correlate.

In experimental infarcts (Figure 1), ^{99m}Tc-PYP images become visible 10–12 hr after infarction. Localization increases and is maximum at 48–72 hr, fades rapidly after 6–7 days, and is almost always absent by 14 days. In humans, positive images have been seen at 10–12 hr (Figure 2), with intensity improving over the next 36–60 hr, but unlike the animal model, some human infarcts remain positive for several weeks. The cause of the continuing positive images is not known. Continued limited cell death or dystrophic calcification in the pericardium or ventricular wall may play a role. Some developing aneurysms have shown uptake of ^{99m}Tc-PYP. If only one study can be performed, we would recommend using the 48-hr postinfarction time interval.

The most common cause for false-negative scintigrams is delay in performance of the imaging procedure until after 6–7 days postinfarction, when the affinity of infarcted tissue for the tracer is rapidly decreasing.

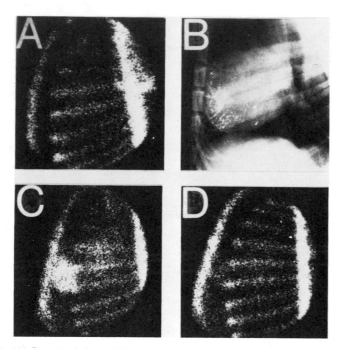

FIGURE 1. (A) Control scintigram (left lateral view) of a dog; (B) X ray of Hg embolus in anterior descending coronary artery causing infarction; (C) scintigram 24 hr postinfarction; (D) scintigram 8 days postinfarction.

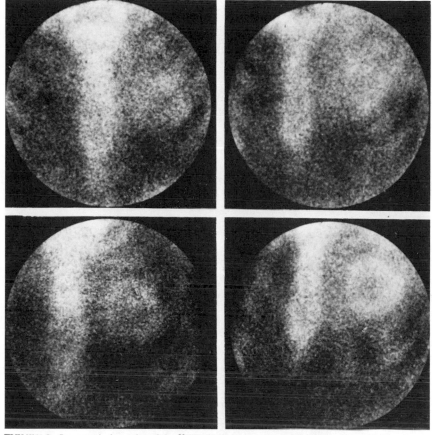

FIGURE 2. Increase in intensity of the ^{99m}Tc-PYP myocardial uptake that occurs with time in most patients with acute transmural myocardial infarctions. Top panels demonstrate the faintly positive ^{99m}Tc-PYP myocardial scintigram approximately 10 hr after myocardial infarction; the lower panels show the more intensely positive scintigram obtained 24 hr later.

The ^{99m}Tc-PYP uptake is dependent on the rate and extent of blood flow to the damaged areas. This leads to a donut configuration in some of the large infarctions (Figure 2).

The technique for imaging acute myocardial infarction is as follows: A dose of 15 mCi ^{99m}Tc tagged to 5 mg stannous pyrophosphate is injected intravenously. (Any phosphate that is stable and has a high tagging efficiency, good blood-clearance properties, and generally gives good bone images should work equally well.) Scintigrams are obtained usually 60–90 min after injection. Postinjection timing needs to fit in the "time window" between blood-pool (early) and marked bone uptake (late). This sometimes varies with age due to differences in renal excretion and bone metabolism. Figure 3 shows sequential

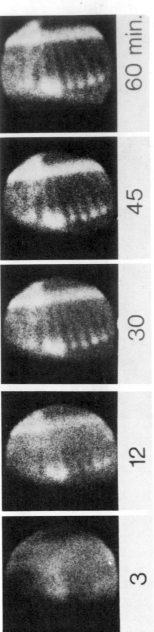
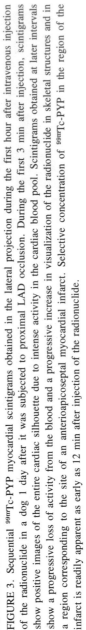

FIGURE 3. Sequential ^{99m}Tc-PYP myocardial scintigrams obtained in the lateral projection during the first hour after intravenous injection of the radionuclide in a dog 1 day after it was subjected to proximal LAD occlusion. During the first 3 min after injection, scintigrams show positive images of the entire cardiac silhouette due to intense activity in the cardiac blood pool. Scintigrams obtained at later intervals show a progressive loss of activity from the blood and a progressive increase in visualization of the radionuclide in skeletal structures and in a region corresponding to the site of an anterioapicoseptal myocardial infarct. Selective concentration of ^{99m}Tc-PYP in the region of the infarct is readily apparent as early as 12 min after injection of the radionuclide.

99mTc-PYP myocardial scintigrams in the lateral projection during the first hour after intravenous injection in a dog 1 day post-LAD occlusion and infarction. Note that the infarction is obscured at 3 min, but is visible as early as 12 min in this young dog with rapid blood clearance. Scintigrams are obtained in the anterior, left lateral, and one or more left anterior oblique projections. Figure 4 demonstrates how an acute infarct can be localized using its rotational relation to the bony landmarks. When rotating from an anterior to a left lateral position, the anterior myocardium rotates with the sternum, while the posterior myocardium rotates away from sternal activity.

Scintigrams are graded from 0 to 4+, depending on the activity over the

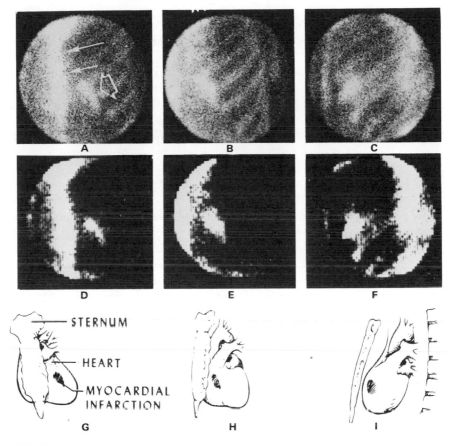

FIGURE 4. Positive (4+) scintigrams of a patient with anterior wall infarction. (A) Anterior view; sternum is indicated by the two smaller arrows with the open arrow pointing to the infarction; (B) 45° left anterior oblique view; (C) left lateral view; (D–F) same as (A–C) after contrast enhancement; (G–I) drawings indicating how area of activity in the myocardium rotates with the anterior wall of the heart.

myocardium. Grading refers to visibility of the suspected lesion and not to size. Zero represents no activity; 1+ indicates minimal activity felt to be in blood pool or chest wall (which is negative with a lower confidence level); 2+, definite activity; and 3+ and 4+ represent increasing degrees of activity within the infarct. Zero and 1+ are considered negative; 2+, 3+, and 4+ are considered positive. This system is arbitrary, but when used clinically, it has shown good correlation with electrocardiographic and enzymatic criteria for determining the presence of infarction. Figure 5 shows examples of zero, 2+, and 4+ myocardial scintigrams. In patients with acute transmural myocardial infarction, about 80% are graded 3+ or 4+ with about 20% being graded 2+. In patients with acute subendocardial infarction, only 40% have 3+ or 4+ scintigrams, and about 60% are graded 2+. Figure 6 shows negative scintigram, while Figure 7 demonstrates ^{99m}Tc-PYP myocardial scintigrams of the different types of transmural infarctions, all graded 4+.

Although computer processing of the images is not usually necessary to visualize an infarct, it is useful in sizing infarctions. Of the three views, the lateral view benefits most from processing. Simple background subtraction and contrast enhancement are all that is usually required, but rib structures can be removed from the images using a one-dimensional, recursive, band-reject digital filter.[17] Sizing of acute anterior and lateral infarcts can be accurately done in dogs.[18,19]

How accurate is this technique? We have found less than 4% false-negative scintigrams when imaging is performed between 1 and 6 days postinfarction. Other groups report 5–10% false-negative results. The exact time of infarction is sometimes difficult to determine, and our ability to do serial imaging probably accounts for the better results. Our false-positive results range from 8–12% if the ECG is used as the standard. Half these patients have "unstable angina pectoris" and could have myocardial necrosis, only detected by scintigraphy. However, future histological correlation is needed. Other groups show false positives ranging from 10 to 20%. Disease processes in which false-positive images might be expected to occur are breast tumors or inflammation, functioning breast parenchyma in premenopausal females, and chest-wall disease of the ribs or muscle. Radioactive ^{99m}Tc-PYP is rapidly cleared by the kidneys and bones, so little pool is present in the heart at 1 hr. If the radiopharmaceutical is poorly tagged, cleared from blood slowly, or if renal disease prevents clearance, a radioactive blood pool in the heart at the time of imaging could give rise to false-positive scintigrams.

This imaging technique represents a simple, noninvasive, and safe procedure for documenting the presence and location of acute myocardial infarction. It does not replace the ECG enzymatic examinations, but adds a new dimension to the physician's understanding of the patient's status. ^{99m}Tc-PYP imaging is particularly valuable in separating old from acute infarcts, detecting

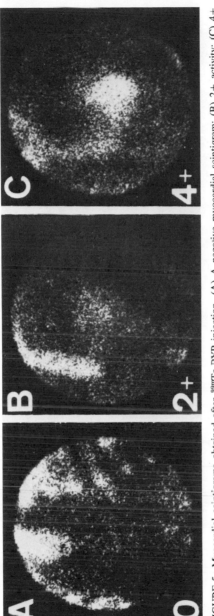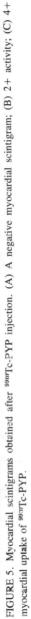

FIGURE 5. Myocardial scintigrams obtained after ^{99m}Tc-PYP injection. (A) A negative myocardial scintigram; (B) 2+ activity; (C) 4+ myocardial uptake of ^{99m}Tc-PYP.

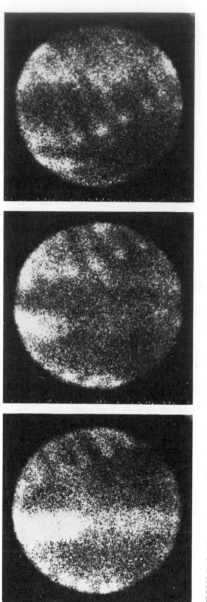

FIGURE 6. Normal myocardial scintigrams. Left to right—anterior, left anterior oblique and left lateral views.

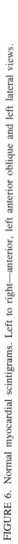

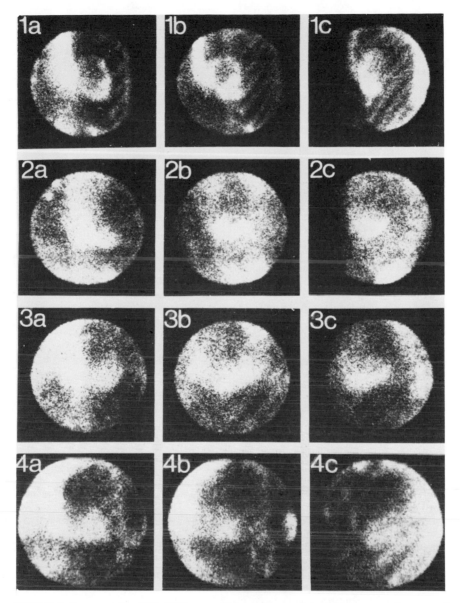

FIGURE 7. Representative ^{99m}Tc-PYP myocardial scintigrams of the different types of transmural myocardial infarction. Vertical columns: (1–4a): Anteroposterior views; (1–4b) anterior oblique views; (1–4c) left lateral views. Horizontal rows: (1a–c) An anterior myocardial infarction; (2a–c) an inferior myocardial infarction; (3a–c) an anterolateral myocardial infarction; (4a–c) a true posterior myocardial infarction.

acute subendocardial infarction, evaluating coronary surgery patients before and after surgery, and sizing anterior and lateral wall infarctions.

References

1. Carr, E. A., Jr., Beierwaltes, W. H., Patno, M. E., Bartlett, J. D., Jr., and Wegst, A. V., The detection of experimental myocardial infarcts by photoscanning, *Amer. Heart J. 64:*650 (1962).
2. Gorten, R. J., Hardy, L. B., McCraw, B. H., Stokes, J. R., and Lumb, G. D., The selective uptake of Hg-203 chormerodrin in experimentally produced myocardial infarcts, *Amer. Heart J. 72:*71 (1966).
3. Malek, P., Vavrejn, B., Ratusky, J., Kronrad, L., and Kolc, J., Detection of myocardial infarction by *in vivo* scanning, *Cardiologia 51:*22 (1967).
4. Hubner, P. J. B., Radioisotopic detection of experimental myocardial infarction using mercury derivatives of fluorescein, *Cardiovasc. Res. 4:*509 (1970).
5. Holma, B. L., Dewanjee, M. K., Idoine, J., Fliegel, C. P., Davis, M. A., Treves, S., and Edlh, P., Detection and localization of experimental myocardial infarction with ^{99m}Tc-tetracycline, *J. Nucl. Med. 14:*595 (1973).
6. Kramer, R. J., Goldstein, R. E., Hirshfeld, J. W., Roberts, W. C., Johnston, G. S., and Epstein, S. E., Accumulation of gallium-67 in regions of acute myocardial infarction, *Amer. J. Cardiol. 33:*861 (1974).
7. Bonte, F. J., Parkey, R. W., Graham, K. D., Moore, J. G., and Stokely, E. M., A new method for radionuclide imaging of myocardial infarcts, *Radiology 110:*473 (1974).
8. Bonte, F. J., Parkey, R. W., Graham, K. D., and Moore, J. G., Distribution of several agents useful in imaging myocardial infarcts, *J. Nucl. Med. 16:*132 (1975.)
9. Parkey, R. W., Bonte, F. J., Meyer, S. L., Atkins, J. M., Curry, G. C., Stokely, E. M., and Willerson, J. T., A new method for radionuclide imaging of acute myocardial infarction in humans, *Circulation 50:*540 (1974).
10. Wilkerson, J. T., Parkey, R. W., Bonte, F. J., Meyer, S. L., and Stokely, E. M., Acute subendocardial myocardial infarction in patients: Its detection by technetium-99*m* stannous pyrophosphate, *Circulation 51:*436 (1975).
11. Willerson, J. T., Parkey, R. W., Bonte, F. J., Meyer, S. L., Atkins, J. M., and Stokely, E. M., Technetium stannous pyrophosphate myocardial scintigrams in patients with chest pain of varying etiology, *Circulation 51:*1046 (1975).
12. D'Agostino, A. W., An electron microscopic study of cardiac necrosis produced by a 9-a-fluorocortisol and sodium phosphate, *Amer. J. Pathol. 45:*633 (1964).
13. D'Agostino, A. W., and Chiga, M., Mitochondrial mineralization in human myocardium, *Amer. J. Clin. Pathol. 53:*820 (1970).
14. Shen, A. C., and Jennings, R. B., Myocardial calcium and magnesium in acute ischemic injury, *Amer. J. Pathol. 67:*417 (1972).
15. Shen, A. C., and Jennings, R. B., Kinetics of calcium accumulation in acute myocardial ischemic injury, *Amer. J. Pathol. 67:*441 (1972).
16. Buja, L. M., Parkey, R. W., Dees, J. H., Stokely, E. M., Harris, R. A., Bonte, F. J., and Willerson, J. T., Morphological correlates of ^{99m}technetium stannous pyrophosphate imaging of acute myocardial infarcts in dogs, *Circulation 52:*596 (1975).
17. Stokely, E. M., Parkey, R. W., Lewis, S. E., Buja, L. M., Bonte, F. J., and Willerson, J. T., Computer processing of ^{99m}Tc-phosphate myocardial scintigrams, in: *Proceedings of IV International Conference on Information Processing Scintigraphy,* Paris (1975).
18. Shames, D. M., Botvinick, E., Lappin, H., Townsend, R., Tybery, J., and Parmley, W.,

Quantitation of myocardial infarct size with Tc-99m pyrophosphate and correlation between myocardial CPK depletion and radionuclide uptake, *J. Nucl. Med. 16:*569 (1975).

19. Stokely, E. M., Buja, L. M., Lewis, S. E., Parkey, R. W., Bonte, F. J., Harris, R. A., Jr., and Willerson, J. T., Sizing of acute myocardial infarcts in dogs with technetium-99m stannous pyrophosphate myocardial scintigrams, *J. Nucl. Med. 71:*1 (1975).

Myocardial Imaging with Thallium-201

Warren R. Janowitz, Denny D. Watson, and Aldo N. Serafini

Introduction

Since myocardial imaging was first described in 1962,[1] many isotopes of rubidium, cesium, nitrogen, potassium, iodine-labeled fatty acids, and others have been utilized as myocardial imaging agents. Their physical and biological characteristics, however, are not well suited to allow myocardial imaging to be done clinically on a routine basis. The ideal agent would be an isotope with a high photon flux with energies that are easily imaged on a gamma camera and with a physical half-life that will permit distribution and a reasonable shelf life of the product, low radiation exposure, and a high myocardial-to-background uptake ratio. Obviously, this agent should also reflect myocardial blood flow accurately.

Work done primarily with potassium-43,[2] rubidium-81,[3] and cesium-129[4] has demonstrated the clinical usefulness of myocardial imaging. Zaret et al.[2] have described much of this work and have also discussed the physiologic basis of myocardial uptake of potassium and some factors that affect the distribution of this intracellular cation within the heart. The primary disadvantage of these agents, however, is that they all emit high-energy photons that make imaging difficult and require special collimation when used with a gamma camera.

The use of thallium as a potassium analogue for myocardial imaging was first suggested by Kawana et al.[5] Thallium-201, which has recently become

WARREN R. JANOWITZ, DENNY D. WATSON, and ALDO N. SERAFINI · Department of Radiology, Baumritter Institute of Nuclear Medicine, Mount Sinai Medical Center, Miami Beach, Florida.

available, has much better physical characteristics for imaging and is currently undergoing evaluation in many centers. Results so far have been promising, and more widespread use of this isotope in the near future seems ensured. The purpose of this paper is to review the pertinent physical and biological properties of thallium-201 and to discuss some of the early clinical results that have been obtained.

Physical Characteristics

Thallium-201 decays by electron capture with a half-life of 73 hr. It emits gamma rays of 135 and 167 keV in 10% abundance. Mercury K X rays of 69 to 83 keV are also emitted in 98% abundance. These photons are easily collimated and imaged with commercially available nuclear instrumentation present in most clinical laboratories.

Thallium-201 is cyclotron-produced in a carrier-free state via the nuclear reaction $^{203}Tl(p, 3n)$ ^{201}Pb. The lead-201 product of this reaction has a half-life of 9.4 hr and is the parent of thallium-201. The lead is chemically separated from the thallium target, allowed to decay for several half-lives, and then separated again with the thallium-201 being obtained in a carrier-free state. Isotopic impurities in the final product include lead-203, thallium-200, and thallium-202, all in very low isotopic abundance.[6]

Thallium-201 is now available from commercial suppliers on an investigational basis and should be more widely available in the near future. The half-life of 73 hr minimizes problems with shipping and distribution and allows a shelf life of 3–4 days.

Biological Behavior

Potassium is the major intracellular cation and in the myocardium is actively transported via the cell-membrane-bound Na^+-K^+ ATPase. Thallium has been shown to behave similarly to potassium. Thus, the sodium- and potassium-activated ATPase can be activated with the substitution of thallium for potassium, and this process does not appear to distinguish between the two elements.[7] The clearance of potassium from the myocardium is faster than that of thallium.[8]

It has also been shown that once inside the cell, thallium is discharged more slowly than potassium.[7] The more rapid turnover of potassium makes the time after injection an important consideration; poor visualization and redistribution can occur if imaging is not done soon after injection. The slower leakage of thallium may be an important advantage when multiple projections are performed that require a longer time for imaging. The problem of redistribution may also be minimized.

Following injection, the disappearance half-time of thallium from the blood is less than 1 min. Myocardial uptake of thallium is rapid, with the peak uptake occurring within 10 min following injection. Studies in animals have shown the myocardial uptake to be approximately $3\frac{1}{2}\%$ of the injected dose 10 min postinjection, which is higher than that obtained with potassium. The relative uptake of the thallium by the heart compared to that of neighboring organs, such as the liver and the lungs, is such that interfering background activity is not a difficult problem, with the relative concentration being optimum for imaging between 10 and 25 min.[7,9]

The distribution of thallium in the heart has been shown to reflect myocardial perfusion. The regional myocardial blood flow, as determined by intracoronary injection of microspheres in dogs, has been compared with the distribution of thallium under conditions of normal flow, partial occlusion, and reactive hyperemia. These studies showed that thallium-201 concentrated in the myocardium in relation to the distribution of regional perfusion. Areas of reactive hyperemia showed increased uptake, though not to the same extent as the increase in microsphere concentration.[8] There is, in this respect, a significant difference between the behavior of thallium and potassium: No significant increase in the concentration of potassium has been observed during reactive hyperemia.[10] Similar correlation of thallium and microsphere distribution has also been obtained in humans.[11]

Although thallium is a toxic compound, the dose required for minimal toxicity has been estimated at 10,000 times the dose required for imaging. Thallium thus appears to have a biological behavior similar to that of potassium in terms of cell uptake, and in some respects it may be superior in that the uptake is higher and leakage from the cell is less than that of potassium. Thus the total accumulation at 10–25 min may be a more accurate reflection of coronary blood flow. There is also no evidence of toxicity with the currently used dosage.

Radiation Dosimetry

Thallium-201 compares favorably in terms of radiation exposure with rubidium-81, cesium-129, and potassium-43. The total body exposure for potassium-43 has been calculated at 0.6 rads/mCi; and thallium-201 has a calculated exposure of 0.07 to 0.24 rads/mCi.[12] These exposures are comparable to those administered in other routine radioisotopic studies.

Clinical Uses of Thallium-201

Technical Aspects. Thallium-201 can easily be imaged on any commercially available scintillation-camera system. The energies are such that a standard low-energy collimator can be used. A recent study comparing a 4000-hole collimator, a high-resolution collimator, and a specially designed converging collimator showed the converging collimator to have the best imaging characteristics. This collimator, however, is currently not available in most nuclear medicine facilities.[13]

After evaluating a number of collimators currently available to us in our institution, a low-energy, high-resolution (10,000-hole) collimator was found to be most satisfactory. The camera is peaked so that counts are accepted from the 69–83 keV X rays. Patients are studied 10–20 min after the intravenous injection of 2 mCi thallium-201 either at rest or following graded treadmill exercise. Anterior, 45° left anterior oblique, 60° left anterior oblique, and left lateral views are obtained. 200,000–300,000 counts/view were obtained, usually taking 2–5 min.

The data, in addition, are collected and stored on line to a commercially available computer for later processing. The capability of image enhancement with a data processor or computer is desirable to suppress background activity. Techniques for quantification of the relative uptake by the heart compared to surrounding lungs have been described; however, due to variable uptake by the background tissues, this technique has limitations, and better methods of quantifying the uptake await development.[14]

In certain instances, such as IHSS, the measurement of wall thickness is important. Unprocessed images have poor resolution of the myocardial wall edges [Figure 1A]; background subtraction, gives some improvement, but still does not give accurate edge positions (Figure 1B). We have used a spatial, double-differentiation technique, which gives a more objective delineation to more of the edge positions, Figures 1C, and D. This technique may be useful in other applications as well.

A typical normal scan is shown in Figure 2A. The anterior projection shows the anterior wall, lateral wall, and apex. Better views of the septum and the anterior, inferior, and posterior walls are obtained in the various LAO and LAT projections. The anterior projection frequently shows some diminished uptake in the apical region, which may cause difficulties in interpretation.

We have found that the lateral view typically has poor resolution and is no longer obtained routinely. This is probably related to the increased distance of the myocardium from the detector with subsequently increased scatter and attenuation.

The 80 keV gamma radiation is attenuated in muscle and blood to a considerable extent with a half-value layer of approximately 3.8 cm. Thus, radiation originating from the posterior myocardial wall is heavily attenuated by absorption in the ventricular chamber and anterior structures. This may be an advantage in visualizing defects in areas of the heart close to the camera since uptake in healthy myocardium behind it will not obscure the defect by a "shine-through" effect. Posterior defects and obese patients may be more difficult to image with this low-energy photon. Rib attenuation will cause a 15–20% reduc-

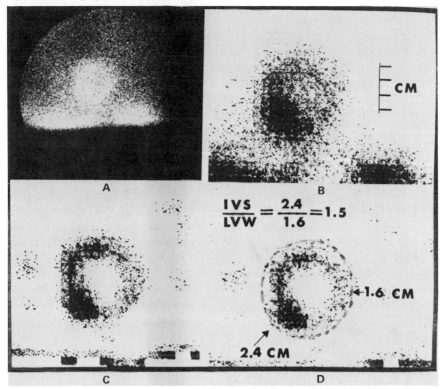

FIGURE 1. (A) Unprocessed thallium image in a patient with IHSS. (B) 30% background suppression. (C) Image processed for edge delineation. (D) Left ventricular wall measurements from processed image with an IVS/LVW ratio of 1.5.

tion in image intensity at the rib positions relative to the intercostal spaces. This is not quite sufficient to show rib shadows on the ordinary scintiphoto images, but enhanced images should be reviewed carefully for possible rib shadow "artifacts."

Thallium-201 Myocardial Scans in Arteriosclerotic Heart Disease

The major applications for thallium-201 myocardial scans appear in the evaluation of arteriosclerotic heart disease, which is the major cause of mortality in the United States. The diagnosis of ASHD in a patient with typical angina pectoris is not difficult. Many patients, however, may have an atypical history, and the diagnosis of ASHD may not be as clearly defined. Although coronary angiography is currently considered to be the definitive procedure for the detection of CAD, it is an invasive procedure involving hospitalization with

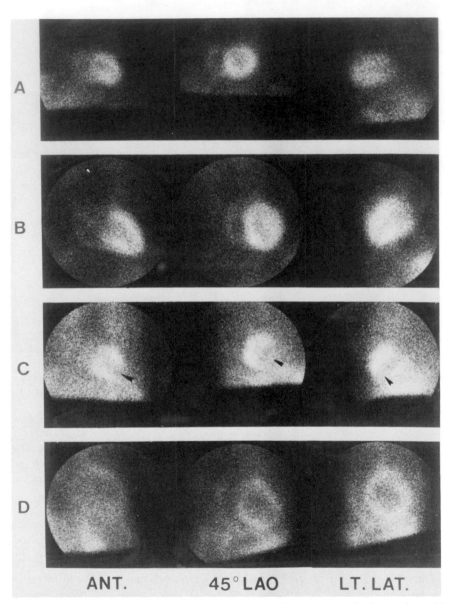

ANT.   45°LAO   LT. LAT.

FIGURE 2. (A) Normal thallium-201 study. (B) Left ventricular hypertrophy in a patient with hypertensive heart disease. (C) Apical - inferior defect in a patient with a documented inferior wall infarct. (D) A 23-year old with a postpartum cardiomyopathy.

some morbidity and mortality and cannot be performed on all patients with chest pain. It also gives no information concerning the microcirculation of the heart. Patients with the so called coronary x disease may have normal angiograms, despite clinical evidence of myocardial ischemia.

A sensitive noninvasive test for the detection of ischemic heart disease is therefore highly desirable. This is commonly done now by the use of ECG monitoring during the performance of various forms of exercise. One form, the Masters two-step test, has been largely replaced by graded bicycle or treadmill exercise. However, even with these techniques, a significant number of false-negative and false-positive results are obtained.

Potassium-43 has been used in conjunction with exercise with some success. Defects at rest have been shown to correspond to old infarcts, whereas defects evident only with stress represent areas of reversible ischemia.

Preliminary studies have also been reported on the use of thallium-201 in conjunction with stress testing; the protocol used is similar to that for potassium-43. Prior to initiating the study, an intravenous line is secured. The thallium-201 is then injected at the point of maximal stress and scintiphotos are obtained 10–15 min postinjection. Several authors have emphasized the need to exercise the patient maximally and to continue with the exercise for approximately 30 sec after injection.

Various investigators have reported on their experience with thallium-201 myocardial scans and arteriosclerotic heart disease. Jambroes et al.,[15] who reported on 24 patients with CAD who had both rest and exercise scans, stated that all CHD patients with positive exercise tests showed defects not present on the resting scan. Ritchie et al.[16] reported on 18 patients with exercise studies, 8 of whom showed new defects with exercise, all of which were associated with coronary artery stenosis >60%. These studies did not comment on the number of false-negative studies. Bailey et al.[17] reported a series of 43 patients with angiographically proved CAD >70%; 33 had abnormal isotope studies either at rest or during exercise and 26 had abnormal rest or exercise ECGs. New thallium defects occurring at exercise, suggesting ischemia, were seen in 26 patients, while abnormal exercise ECGs were seen in 14. Of 21 patients with single-vessel disease, the scans were abnormal in 15 and ECGs detected 8; 18 patients with double- or triple-vessel disease were detected by both techniques. Their impression was that thallium was more sensitive than exercise ECGs in the diagnosis of CAD, especially in single vessel disease.

The experience at our institution with exercise scans has been similar to that previously reported. We have, however, seen several patients with single-vessel disease, positive exercise tests, and negative thallium scan. Figure 3 shows the anterior and 45° LAO thallium scans, the ECG at the time of injection, and the cineangiogram of one of these patients who had a 75% occlusion of the left circumflex and first diagonal branch of the left coronary artery. Another patient

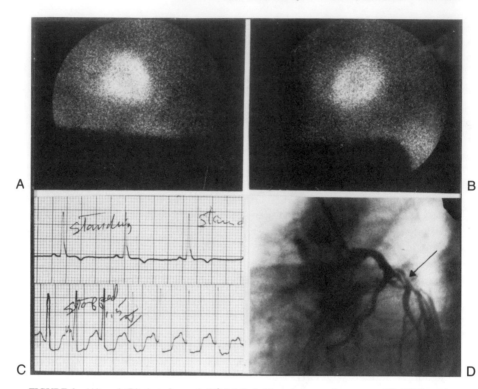

FIGURE 3. (A) and (B) Anterior and 45° LAO thallium images after stress. (C) ECG tracings prior to exercise and at the time of injection of thallium-201. (D) Coronary angiogram demonstrating 75% occlusion of circumflex branch, left coronary artery.

with a positive exercise ECG, single-vessel disease, and >75% occlusion of the LAD had normal rest and exercise thallium studies. We therefore feel that though thallium may be more sensitive than exercise electrocardiogram, the presence of a normal scan does not exclude significant CAD. This is in contrast to the report of Zaret et al.,[18] using potassium-43, in which positive exercise tests with normal potassium-43 scans were associated with normal angiograms.

Thallium-201 Myocardial Scans in Myocardial Infarction

Thallium-201 imaging done at rest may also be useful in the detection of acute myocardial infarction. Studies with induced infarcts in dogs have shown, using thallium, that defects correlate well with areas of infarction and of increased technetium-99m pyrophosphate uptake[19] in acute infarcts. It has also been used to diagnose infarction in patients with left bundle branch block.[20] Some groups feel that thallium-201 may be more accurate than technetium-99m pyrophosphate in the diagnosis and localization of acute infarcts.[21] The sizing of infarcts early in the course of myocardial infarction may allow more vigorous treatment to be directed to those patients whose scans indicate large areas of infarction and who are more likely to develop problems. An advantage of thallium-201 is that the study can be done within hours of the infarct rather than the 12–48 hr needed for the technetium-99m pyrophosphate scans to turn positive. Unfortunately, thallium cannot distinguish old from new infarcts. Figure 1C shows an apical-inferior defect in a patient with a documented inferior wall infarction.

Our experience has also shown that thallium-201 scanning at rest is useful in the precatheterization evaluation of patients who are candidates for coronary bypass surgery—large defects at rest have been shown to be associated with areas of akinesis and scarring. These patients usually have significantly lower ejection fractions and have an increased surgical risk. Figure 4 shows the thallium images and intrinsically gated technetium-99m HSA systolic and diastolic images in a patient with a large area of apical akinesis. This was confirmed at catheterization, and the patient was not felt to be a good surgical candidate.

Although this work is preliminary, the use of combined isotopic studies using thallium, gated systolic and diastolic images, and $C^{15}O_2$ inhalation for ejection fraction and regurgitant fraction enables us to obtain a fairly complete evaluation of a patient's cardiac status. Those patients with diffuse ventricular dysfunction can be differentiated from those with potentially surgically correctable diseases. Catheterization can then be avoided in some patients.

Other Uses

Thallium has also been useful in other nonischemic forms of heart disease. For example, left ventricular hypertrophy can be detected [see Figure 2B]. Also, uses in asymmetric septal hypertrophy[22] (see Figure 1) right ventricular hypertrophy,[23] and sarcoid heart disease[24] have been reported. The differentiation between septal hypertrophy due to IHSS and that due to right ventricular hypertrophy can be made.

Figure 1D shows the thallium image of a patient with a postpartum cardiomyopathy. This patient died several weeks after having been scanned and autopsy confirmed a large dilated heart without infarction as suggested by the image.

Summary

In conclusion, it appears that thallium-201:
1. Has biological behavior similar to potassium and in some ways superior to it.

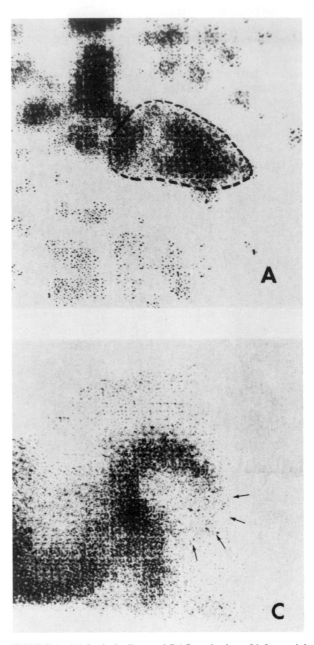

FIGURE 4. (A) Intrinsically gated RAO projection of left ventricle
akinesis; (C) thallium scintiphoto showing large apical defect; (D),

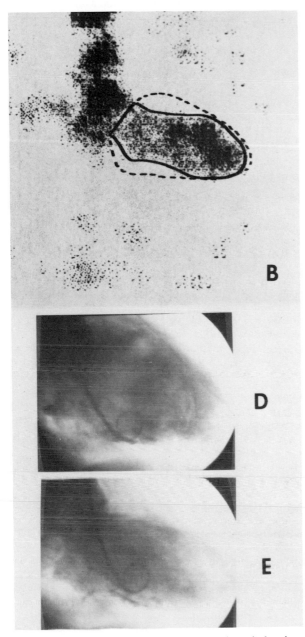

in diastole; (B) systolic image showing large anterior-apical region of
(E) diastolic and systolic left ventricular cineangiogram.

2. Has physical properties that are the best of the currently available isotopes for myocardial imaging.
3. Is more sensitive than exercise ECGs in the diagnosis of ASHD.
4. Is very accurate in the detection, localization, and possibly the sizing of acute infarcts.
5. May be useful as a screening procedure, in conjunction with other isotopic studies, prior to cardiac catheterization to evaluate the extent of myocardial dysfunction.
6. Is useful in the diagnosis of other cardiac diseases.

More work is needed to assess its role in these situations accurately and to establish the incidence of false-positive and false-negative tests; however, thallium-201 at present seems to be the most valuable myocardial-imaging agent available.

References

1. Carr, E. A., Jr., Beirwaltes, W. H., Wegit, A. V., and Bartlett, J. D. Jr., Myocardial scanning with Rubidium-86, *J. Nucl. Med. 3:*76 (1962).
2. Zaret, B. L., Strauss, H. W., Martin, N. D., Wells, H. P. Jr., and Flamm, M. D., Jr., Noninvasive regional myocardial perfusion with radioactive potassium: Study of patients at rest, with exercise and during angina pectoris, *N. Engl. J. Med. 288:*809 (1973).
3. Berman, D. S., Salel, A. F., DeNardo, G. L., and Mason, D. T., Noninvasive detection of regional myocardial ischemia using Rb-81 and the scintillation camera, *Circulation 52:*619 (1975).
4. Romhilt, D. W., Adolph, R. J., Dodd, V. J., Levenson, N. I., August, L. S., Nishiyamas, H., and Berke, R. A., Cesium-129 myocardial scintigraphy to detect myocardial infarction, *Circulation 48:*1242 (1973).
5. Kawana, M., Krizeh, H., Porter, J., Lathrop, K. A., Charleston, D., and Harper, P. V., Use of ^{199}Tl as a potassium analogue in scanning, *J. Nucl. Med. 11:*333 (1970).
6. Lebowitz, E., Green, M. W., Fairchild, R., Bradley-Moore, P. R., Atkins, H. L., Ansari, A. N., Richards, P., and Belgrave, E., Thallium-201 for medical use, I., *J. Nucl. Med. 16:*151 (1975).
7. Gehring, P. J., and Hammond, P. B., The interrelationship between thallium and potassium in animals, *J. Pharm. Exp. Ther. 155:*187 (1967).
8. Strauss, H. W., Harrison, K., Tangan, J. K., Lebowitz, E., and Pitt, B., Thallium-201 for myocardial imaging, *Circulation 511:*641 (1975).
9. Bradley-Moore, P. R., Lebowitz, E., Greene, M. W., Atkins, H. L., and Ansari, A. N., Thallium-201 for medical use. II. Biologic behavior, *J. Nucl. Med. 16:*156 (1975).
10. Prokop, E. K., Strauss, H. W., Shaw, J., Pitt, B., and Wagner, H. N., Jr., Comparison of regional myocardial perfusion determined by ionic potassium-43 to that determined by microspheres, *Circulation 50:*978 (1974).
11. Ritchie, J. L., Hamilton, G. W., Williams, D. L., English, M. T., and Leibowitz, E., Myocardial imaging with thallium-201-correlation with intracoronary macroaggregated albumin imaging, *Circulation* (Supp II.) *52:*231 (1975).
12. Feller, P. A., and Sodd, V. J., Dosimetry of your heart-imaging radionuclides: K-43, Rb-81, Cs-129, and Tl-201, *J. Nucl. Med. 16:*1070 (1975).
13. Groch, M. W., and Lewis, G. K., Thallium-201: Scintillation camera imaging considerations, *J. Nucl. Med. 17:*142 (1976).

14. Rouleau, J., Griffith, L., Strauss, H. W., and Pitt, B., Detection of diffuse coronary artery disease by quantification of Thallium-201 myocardial images, *Circulation* (Suppl. II) *52:* (1975).

15. Jambroes, G., vanRigk, P. P., vendeBerg, C. J. M., and deGraaf, C. N., Thallium-201 rest and exercise scintigraphy in patients with coronary heart disease, *Circulation* (Suppl. II) *52:*111 (1975).

16. Ritchie, J. L., Trobaugh, G. B., Hamilton, G. W., Weaver, D., Williams, D. L., and Gould, K. L., Rest and exercise myocardial imaging with Thallium-201—Correlation with EKG, coronary anatomy, and left ventricular function, *Amer. J. Cardiol. 37:*166 (1976).

17. Bailey, I. K., Griffith, S. C., Strauss, H. W., and Pitt, B., Detection of coronary artery disease and myocardial ischemia by electrocardiography and myocardia perfusion scanning with Thallium-201, *Amer. J. Cardiol. 37:*118 (1976).

18. Zaret, B. L., Stenson, R. E., Martin, N. D., Strauss, H. W., Wells, H. P., McGowan, R. L., and Flamm, M. D., Potassium-43 myocardial perfusion scanning for the noninvasive evaluation of points with false-positive exercise tests, *Circulation 48:*1234 (1973).

19. Buja, L. M., Parkey, R. W., Stokely, E. M., Bonte, F. J., and Willerson, J. T., Pathophysiology of Tc-99m stannous pyrophosphate and thallium-201 scintigraphy of canine acute myocardial infarctions, *Circulation* (Suppl. II) *52:*51 (1975).

20. Wackers, F. J., Lie, K. I., Sokole, E., Schoot, J. V. D., Durrer, D., and Wellens, H. J., Thallium-201 for localization of acute myocardial infarction in the presence of left bundle branch block, *Circulation* (Suppl. II) *52:*54 (1975).

21. Schelbert, H., Henning, H., Righetti, A., Ashburn, W., and O'Rourke, R., Relative sensitivity of Tc-99m pyrophosphate and thallium-201 for diagnosing acute myocardial infarction, *Amer. J. Cardiol. 37:*170 (1976).

22. Bulkley, B. H., Rouleair, J., Strauss, H. W., and Pitt, B., Idiopathic hypertropic subaortic stenosis: detection by thallium-201 myocardial perfusion imaging, *N. Engl. J. Med. 293:*1113 (1975).

23. Stevens, R. M., Baird, M. G., Fuhrmann, C. F., Rouleau, J., Summer, W. R., Strauss, H. W., and Pitt, B., Detection of right ventricular hypertrophy by thallium-201 myocardial perfusion imaging, *Circulation* (Suppl. II) *52:*243 (1975).

24. Bulkley, B. H., Rouleau, J., Strauss, H. W., and Pitt, B., Sarcoid heart disease: Diagnosis by thallium-201 myocardial perfusion imaging, *Amer. J. Cardiol. 37:*125 (1976).

Part IV·Evaluation of Ventricular Function

Functional Aspects of Myocardial and Valvular Disease: Clinical Correlations

Frank J. Hildner

A Cardiologist's Approach to the Cardiac Patient

An accurate and complete evaluation of heart function requires a systematic approach. The most commonly used method is composed of five logical steps. The first two elements are a satisfactory history and a thorough physical examination, which in the vast majority of cases permit at least a preliminary diagnosis to be made. The third step in the evaluation of a cardiac patient is the use of noninvasive techniques to define cardiac function. In the remote past, this was limited almost exclusively to the ECG, but in recent years, development of the phonocardiogram, vectorcardiogram, and especially the echocardiogram and noninvasive techniques, such as systolic time intervals and exercise stress, have permitted far more accurate and precise diagnoses. The fourth step includes the chest radiograph, which permits overall estimation of the cardiac and individual chamber sizes. The fifth and last step in this approach to cardiac diagnosis is cardiac catheterization. This technique has classically been reserved for the more difficult cases. It also serves as a foundation for all other diagnostic efforts. During the past ten years however, marked improvement in equipment technology and development of safer new techniques have permitted catheterization to be employed far more frequently.

Where do radionuclide techniques fit into the scheme of the cardiologist's approach to a patient? We have learned that nuclide angiography permits

FRANK J. HILDNER · Department of Medicine, University of Miami School of Medicine, Miami, Florida; and Department of Cardiology, Mount Sinai Medical Center, Miami Beach, Florida.

evaluation of the systolic ejection fraction and possibly even systolic or diastolic ventricular volumes. We have also learned that left ventricular "pump function" can be estimated by radionuclide techniques and that it is possible to estimate cardiac output and myocardial contractility from radionuclide studies. It is worthwhile to ask now whether these techniques are giving the answers cardiologists desire or whether they are simply other laboratory procedures that give truthful information of little clinical significance. As a matter of fact, information such as ventricular volumes, ejection fraction, circumferential fiber shortening, and heart rate derived from newer radionuclide techniques is precisely the information the cardiologist should be utilizing in the evaluation of heart function. Unfortunately, it seems that many cardiologists do not realize this and therefore do not appreciate the value they have potentially at hand. While this is a very strong statement, I believe a short review of cardiovascular diagnostic techniques will clarify the issue.

Cardiac Diagnosis—Historical Aspects

Before catheterization, the cardiologist knew very little about the internal functioning of human heart and its relationship to clinical situations, and application of principles from animal studies was not always satisfactory. The first step toward better diagnosis came when right heart catheterizations permitted measurement of the right heart pressures and the cardiac output. Reflected left atrial pressure from the wedge position inaugurated intensive study of left ventricular hemodynamics. Shortly thereafter, left heart catheterization with the full application of angiocardiography brought about a revolution that permitted careful estimation of valve function and permitted application of openheart surgery. Even at this point, the cardiologists relied chiefly on individual chamber pressures, transvalvular pressure differences, and cardiac output as the major indicators of cardiac performance. One was able to estimate roughly the ability of the ventricle to squeeze, and rudimentary estimates concerning segmental contraction abnormalities were rendered. In due course many interventions were added to the catheterization procedure, provoking responses from the heart that permitted further evaluation of residual function. Bicycle ergometric studies, simple leg-raising, and hand grip induced a change in resting state that could be quantitated and, in some cases, permitted more accurate evaluation of the cardiac status than could be obtained by measurement of resting function alone. Other interventions, such as atrial pacing and the infusion of drugs, such as epinephrine, angiotensin, and isoproterinol, provoked other responses, all of which permitted further evaluation of the patient's cardiac status. While all of these permitted somewhat better evaluation of the ventricular functional status, it was the application of mechanical principles to the cardiac physiology that has revolutionized the practice of cardiology in all its areas, including the office, the hospital, and the intensive care unit. Rather than simply using the heart rate, cardiac output, and left ventricular end-diastolic pressure as end products, we now use them as substrate to develop derived data, which paint a clearer picture of cardiac function and define cardiac status much more accurately.

Modern Cardiac Catheterization

While we speak of catheterization as the tool that has so successfully paced the advancement of cardiologic practice, it is truly angiocardiography that is the central focus of our attention. Only through angiocardiography has the clinician been able to evaluate ventricular volumes, ejection fraction, the ability of the muscle to contract, thickness of the myocardial muscle, the rate of change of myocardial fiber shortening, and evaluation of areas of poor or abnormal contraction. These values, obtained properly and combined with other parameters, such as left ventricular stroke-work index, left ventricular end-diastolic pressure, cardiac output, and rate of rise of the ventricular pressure, when normalized among a large series of hearts, permit an accurate evaluation of the overall functional state of the myocardium. Thus, what was only a left ventricular end-diastolic pressure before, when compared to a calculated value of stroke work (cardiac output times the aortic pressure times the weight of blood) now becomes a ventricular-function curve, which permits accurate estimation of the ability of the heart to do its job. This approach to cardiac function has been of extreme practical value in caring for the acute cardiac problems in the intensive care unit. We have learned that the left-ventricular filling pressure, derived from a right heart catheter in a wedge position in the lungs or from a balloon occlusive device, permitting measurement of reflected left atrial pressure, can be used as an indication of the functional integrity of the left ventricle. A pressure over 20 mm Hg indicates loss of ventricular competence, whereas a pressure well below 10 mm Hg may indicate that the ventricle is functioning inefficiently because of a lack of volume or a lack of fluid return to the heart. These critical determinations have been developed from the meticulous comparison of left-ventricular physiologic events during the various stages of clinical cardiac sufficiency and failure. The optimum stretching of the myocardial fiber, according to Starling's law of the heart, results in the development of a left-ventricular filling pressure of certain magnitude. The ejection fraction by itself or in combination is similarly useful clinically. It is certain that this approach to cardiac function has resulted in a revolution in the broad field of cardiology today.

It is unfortunate that many cardiologists do not fully appreciate the advances that have been made. For example, at the time of cardiac catheterization for coronary arteriography, LV angiography and derived measurements are omitted.

Many cardiologists fail to appreciate the value of left ventricular angiocardiography and the measurements that may be derived therefrom. Similarly, many cardiologists prefer to treat an acute myocardial infarction complicated by hypotension, shock, or other profound hemodynamic alteration without the use of a Swan-Ganz catheter in the pulmonary artery or even arterial or venous lines. It is unfortunate that many cardiologists still rely on the ECG and chest X ray as prime techniques for cardiovascular diagnosis without the use of even the more common, though limited, applicability of echocardiography and similar noninvasive pursuits. And while treadmill exercise has improved the yield of accurate diagnoses as compared to the Master's two-step test, many physicians are willing to accept it as conclusive, failing to understand its limitations so adequately demonstrated frequently by cardiac catheterization and coronary arteriography. The point to be made here is that information derived from any single determination of a single cardiac variable has very little value. This is especially true of such previously important single parameters as LVEDP, cardiac output, vectorcardiogram, echocardiogram, ECG, and treadmill testing. If one were to prescribe a list of determinants, which when used as a group and in combination should adequately describe ventricular function to the best of our ability at this time in history, one would undoubtedly include the following:

1. Heart rate
2. LVEDP
3. Ventricular volumes
4. Ejection fraction
5. Stroke-work index
6. A measure of myocardial contractility (such as circumferential fiber-shortening velocity)
7. Compliance

Practical Application of Radionuclide Technology

Radionuclide techniques that are currently available or soon to be in widespread use are able to provide a large number of the determinants that will permit evaluation of cardiac function. It is possible that very soon radionuclide technology will advance its capabilities and provide efficient means for the determination of ventricular volumes, ejection fraction, and myocardial contraction velocity. These left-ventricular determinants, when combined with a right heart catheter recording the left-ventricular filling pressure, which is a rough guide to the LVEDP, may provide a clue to the functional capacity of the left ventricle and permit evaluation of severe left ventricular dysfunction in an acutely ill patient without the necessity of left ventricular angiography. While this is still theoretical and will require a great deal of intensive investigation and clinical correlative study, the possibility exists and is almost immediately at hand.

One need not look to the future to find practical applications of radionuclide techniques. Those that are available today are of value and should be employed in practical situations. Therefore, these techniques should be utilized in the most advantageous manner. As with other cardiovascular investigations, random radionuclide examinations are less beneficial than when they are combined with another determination, e.g., a Swan-Ganz catheter in the pulmonary artery. The recording camera must be available at the patient's bedside, particularly in the intensive care unit. In the patient who has chest pain, ventricular size may not be particularly important, although a very low ejection fraction may deter some surgeons from the operation. If ventricular-size determinations made from radioangiograms are truly reliable, this may be a worthwhile screening technique in many instances. Similarly, evaluation of ventricular size or ejection fraction in patients with valvular disease may not be important if done on a single preoperative basis. However, this evaluation assumes prognostic value if serial postoperative determinations show a distinct change from the preoperative one. It is important for the radionuclide study to be available where other techniques are not available, such as in the intensive care unit where angiocardiography is usually not possible. It is important for the radionuclide study to avoid duplication of results obtainable in a more precise and accurate manner, such as cardiac catheterization. However, if the radionuclide study is able to furnish an advantage over other techniques, such as repeated studies after a given event, its ultimate usefulness and value will have been established.

Techniques for Heart–Lung Imaging

D. D. Watson, A. N. Serafini, J. J. Greenberg,
and A. J. Gilson

Introduction

Color labeling and retrospective time-interval selection have been used to produce scintiphotographic images of the central blood flow in conjunction with the
radionuclide cardiac flow study. The images are formed by integrating over time
intervals, chosen retrospectively to include the entire right heart, lung, or left
heart (levo) phase of the radionuclide bolus transit. This provides improved
statistical delineation of the images, and also tends to produce an intensity
modulation inversely proportional to the local volume flow rate. Selected composite images may then be recorded on Polaroid color film through colored filters
to obtain color contrast between adjacent or overlapping areas of the images.
Intensity modulation is used in the conventional manner within each
monochrome image. The resultant image is easily interpretable and more inform-
ative than conventional sequential scintiphotos.

Methods

Patients are placed supine beneath a scintillation camera interfaced to a
minicomputer system. A sheet source containing ^{99m}Tc is placed beneath the
patient, and the patient is positioned by viewing the cardiac silhouette on a
persistence oscilloscope. A transmission image of the cardiac silhouette is then

D. D. WATSON, A. N. SERAFINI, J. J. GREENBERG, and A. J. GILSON · Department of
Radiology, Baumritter Institute of Nuclear Medicine, Mount Sinai Medical Center, Miami Beach,
Florida.

recorded. The sheet source is removed, and 10–15 mCi ^{99m}Tc pertechnetate is injected as a bolus. Serial images are recorded by the camera and computer at the rate of 1 frame/sec. Computer images are generated by summing over time intervals selected for the individual study and displayed on a CRT in a conventional 64×64 matrix.

Time intervals for the image formation are chosen to extend, e.g., from the time of bolus arrival in the left heart throughout the clearance phase until the time of bolus recirculation. Stated more simply, the image is integrated throughout the levo phase. Right heart images are similarly integrated throughout the right heart phase. When this is done, each picture element contains a number of counts N_i in proportion to the integral of the radionuclide indicator concentration curve $C_i(t)$ corresponding to the region of that picture element. That is,

$$N_i \approx \int C_i(t)dt \tag{1}$$

The well-known principle of indicator-dilution is

$$F = \frac{Q}{\int C(t)dt} \tag{2}$$

Elimination of $\int C(t)dt$ between Eq. (1) and Eq. (2) yields the following result:

$$N_i \approx \frac{Q}{F_i} \tag{3}$$

where F_i represents the local rate of flow within the area associated with the ith picture element. This reasoning, while only approximate, points out that images formed by integrating over the entire bolus transit time tend to have an intensity that is *inversely* related to the rate of flow. The image intensity will be greater when the flow rate is lower. This effect will be illustrated in the following examples.

In the examples given (Figure 1), only two colors (blue-green and yellow-orange) are employed. Each color is also intensity modulated. The use of more colors in more vivid hues is more spectacular, but has been found to add no significant information. The colors illustrated can be easily obtained through filters from any standard oscilloscope phosphor.

Discussion

If some device to select and form scintiphotographic images is available, the methods described above are quite simple and inexpensive. Aneurysm of the

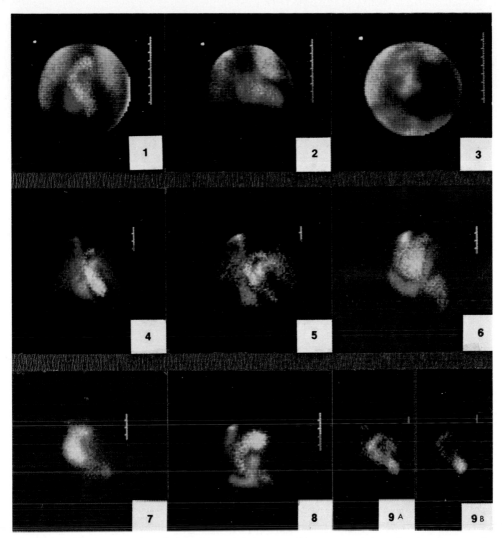

FIGURE 1. (1) A composite of right heart, left heart, and lung transmission, showing the smooth-bordered gap between the heart and the lungs, which is typical of pericardial effusion; (2) a similar composite; in this case, the enlarged cardiac silhouette is seen to be due entirely to a dilated left ventricle; (3) a composite showing the effects of a solid pericardial mass; the heart is compressed and slightly displaced; (4) an overlapped image of the right heart and the left heart with a normal thickness of the ventricular wall; (5) an overlapped image demonstrating concentrically increased left-ventricular wall thickness; the patient was found to have aortic stenosis with left-ventricular hypertrophy; (6) an overlapped image demonstrating an aneurysm of the ascending aorta; there is also an aneurysm near the apex of the left ventricle; (7) an integrated left heart image demonstrating a dissecting aneurysm of the ascending aorta, starting from the aortic valve plane; increased brightness in the region of the aneurysm is due to the inverse flow-rate-intensity modulation discussed in the text; (8) an overlapped image demonstrating an aneurysm at the arch of the aorta; (9a) a left heart image formed by a short integration time in the early levo phase; (9b) the same heart as in (9a), but with a longer time integration demonstrating reduced blood flow in the region of an apical aneurysm of the left ventricle.

ventricles or great vessels, pericardial effusion, mediastinal masses, and myocardial wall thickness are more readily appreciated when displayed in this manner than from conventional sequential scintiphotos.

Acknowledgment

This work was supported by USPHS Grant HL-15780.

Noninvasive Measurement of Left-Ventricular Performance Utilizing an Anger Camera–Left-Ventricular Ejection Fraction

William L. Ashburn, Heinrich R. Schelbert,
Gary Brock, Hartmut Henning, John W. Verba,
Naomi P. Alazraki, and Allen D. Johnson

Introduction

During the past several years and in cooperation with our cardiology colleagues, we have attempted to perfect a method of determining left-ventricular ejection fraction that can be applied in the evaluation of patients with left-ventricular dysfunction. It might be helpful to remember that ejection fraction is one method of estimating left-ventricular performance and describes the percentage of LV blood that is ejected with each systolic contraction (ejection fraction equals stroke volume/end-diastolic volume).

Recent reports[1-4] have shown that it is possible to determine several parameters of left-ventricular performance, such as end-diastolic and stroke volume as well as ejection fraction by analysis of the pattern of transit of a ^{99m}Tc bolus through the left ventricle. This report will describe in detail our method of calculating left-ventricular ejection fraction from data obtained with a scintillation camera. This method is based on the original work of Van Dyke et al.,[5] in

WILLIAM L. ASHBURN, HEINRICH R. SCHELBERT, GARY BROCK, HARTMUT HENNING, JOHN W. VERBA, NAOMI P. ALAZRAKI, and ALLEN D. JOHNSON · Department of Radiology and the Department of Medicine, University of California Medical Center, San Diego, California. Work supported in part by NHLBI grant HL-17682.

which the cyclical high-frequency components of the LV time activity occurring with each heartbeat are analyzed.

Recordings are made with the scintillation-camera detector in the 20° right anterior oblique position. Data are recorded on magnetic tape in a digital ("list") format for subsequent computer analysis. Approximately 10–15 mCi ^{99m}Tc albumin (or pertechnetate) is injected as a bolus of less than 1 ml either into the superior vena cava in patients studied in the cardiac catheterization laboratory, into a peripheral arm vein in patients with acute myocardial infarction, or in severely ill patients through a Swan-Ganz catheter positioned in the pulmonary artery. The advantage of labeled albumin is that following the initial circulation of the tracer, gated blood-pool imaging in several projections can be accomplished.[6,7] Alternatively, tracers, such as ^{99m}Tc pyrophosphate, can be substituted. Thus, after the initial transit of the bolus through the left ventricle has been recorded, acute "infarct" imaging can be performed in 1–2 hr.[8]

On replay of the raw scintillation-camera data, curve analysis can be performed on a small dedicated computer (e.g., General Electric MED-2). Data analysis consists of first assigning a region of interest (ROI) corresponding to the LV chamber and second, a horseshoe-shaped ROI, roughly corresponding to the immediately surrounding noncardiac structures, which is used to compensate for "background" activity.

The assignment of these ROIs is illustrated in Figure 1, which shows the LV and the aortic arch (A) and the two ROIs corresponding to the left ventricle and the background area (B). The background ROI curve (not shown) is normalized under automatic computer control by the ratio of memory locations assigned in the background ROI to the number of memory locations assigned in the LV ROI. Curve correction is accomplished by subtracting, point for point, the background curve from the raw LV curve. The resulting time–activity curve (C) is displayed at 1 sec/point and demonstrates two peaks. The first corresponds to the passage of the bolus through the superimposed right ventricle and the second is coincident with its passage through the left ventricle. These data can be used for calculating cardiac output (when ^{99m}Tc albumin is used) and/or pulmonary mean transit time and pulmonary blood volume if cardiac output is known. The operator then instructs the computer to produce a higher resolution display of the second peak, which corresponds to the transit of radioactivity through the left ventricle and consists of 25 points/sec, i.e., 40 msec/point (D).

The cyclical changes in count rate during each cardiac cycle are best appreciated by examining a computer printout of a typical LV time-activity curve (Figure 2). Cyclical peaks and valleys are seen throughout the curve: The high points in each cycle correspond to the LV count rate at end-diastole and the low points, to end-systole. Since mixing of the radioactive bolus with the blood of the left ventricle is assumed to be complete at the time of maximum count rate within the left ventricle, only the first 3 or 4 cardiac cycles (between the arrows) on the

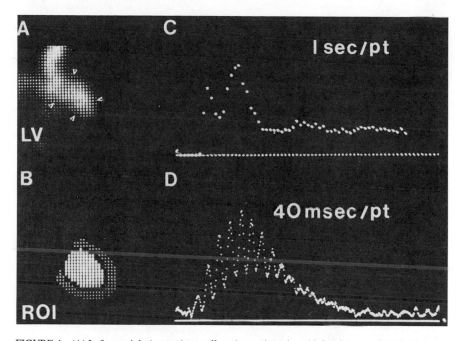

FIGURE 1. (A) Left ventricle (arrows) as well as the aortic arch and left atrium are visualized during the passage of a ⁹⁹Tc bolus through these structures as imaged in the right anterior oblique projection and recorded in a 64×64 data matrix. (B) Regions of interest (ROI) are assigned to correspond to the left ventricle (brighter dots) as well as the surrounding background zone (darker dots). (C) After correction for background contributions (see text), a time–activity curve is derived during the transit of the radioactive bolus through the LV ROI. The first of the two peaks corresponds to the arrival of the bolus in the superimposed right ventricle; the second peak, to its appearance in the left ventricle. Each point represents counts accumulated for 1 sec. (D) A higher (time) resolution display of the second (LV) peak in the preceding panel. Cyclical changes in count rate with each cardiac cycle can be recognized when the curve points are displayed at 25 samples/sec (40 msec/point).

downslope of the curve are used for ejection-fraction determination. Experience has shown that if the calculations are made using data on the upslope before mixing, ejection-fraction values are routinely too high. [LV ejection fraction is derived by dividing the difference in count rate between end-diastole (peak) and end-systole (valley) by the count rate at end-diastole. Then these values are averaged over 3–4 consecutive cardiac cycles.]

Examination of a typical dilution curve discloses a statistical problem in that counts/40 msec rarely exceed 100. This might seem surprising, considering that maximum count rates within the entire scintillation-camera field of view average approximately 15,000 counts/sec when 10–15 mCi ⁹⁹ᵐTc is injected, which, of course, depends to a considerable extent on the type of collimator used. Thus in order to place less reliance on individual high and low 40-msec values, we

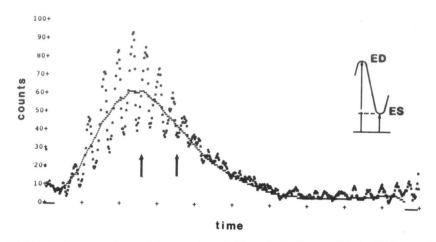

FIGURE 2. Computer printout of the curve shown in Figure 1. (D) Counts within the LV for each 40 msec are plotted against time (2 sec between marks). Only the first three or four cardiac cycles (between arrows) following the maximum count rate are analyzed. The high points of each cardiac cycle correspond to end-diastole (ED), and the following valley to end-systole (ES). The ejection fraction is calculated by ED−ES/ED.

employ a method using the root-mean-square derivation of amplitude of sinusoidal fluctuations in data as the basis of our analysis. We assume that changes in the LV volume (and therefore in the count rate) during each cardiac cycle can be approximated by sinusoidal function. Accordingly, an average curve is fit by the computer to the data (indicated by the dotted line in Figure 2). The deviations of the fluctuating raw data from the average curve are determined and the root-mean square, i.e., the square root of the mean of the squares of the variations, is calculated. Then standard sine-wave analysis is employed, which states that the amplitude (peak height) of a sinusoidal variation is equal to the square root of two times the root mean square. Thus, the difference between the count rates at end-diastole and end-systole (stroke volume) is expressed as two times the square root of two times the root mean square. By this method, therefore, all the data points during each cardiac cycle (rather than single high and low 40-msec values) are considered in the calculation, thereby considerably improving the statistical reliability of the determination.

In order to compare the accuracy of the radionuclide method for determining ejection fraction with X-ray contrast biplane cineangiography, 20 patients with suspected ischemic heart disease, excluding patients with valvular heart disease, were evaluated by both techniques in the cardiac catheterization laboratory. Close agreement between the radionuclide method and biplane cineangiography was demonstrated with a correlation coefficient of $r = 0.94$. The ejection fractions ranged from a high of 0.80 to a low of 0.20 (normal in our laboratory is 0.52).

To test the ability of different observers in using the interactive computer routine, two physicians and one physicist independently determined ejection fractions in 6 consecutive patients. The agreement was very close in each case, which suggests that the technique can be easily learned by relatively inexperienced persons.

One of the potential sources of error using this technique is incorrect assignment of the background ROI. When no background ROI is assigned, average ejection fractions are lower than those determined by cineangiography. On the other hand, when the background ROI is assigned as a ring completely surrounding the left ventricle, including a portion of the aortic arch, average ejection fractions are consistently too high. The correct background ROI has been empirically determined to be a semicircle that does not include any portion of the left ventricle nor extend into the aortic arch.

Similarly, the precise requirements of LV ROI assignment have been studied. When the LV is too small, ejection fractions tend to be falsely high. If the LV ROI includes a portion of the aortic arch, ejection fractions are too low. However, even if the LV ROI tends to be slightly too large, values do not differ significantly and agree closely with biplane cineangiographic determinations. This probably reflects the fact that radioactivity extending slightly beyond the apparent LV outline nonetheless represent valid time-dependent data.

Clinical experience with this nontraumatic method of determining ejection fraction suggests that it can be used successfully in the serial assessment of LV performance in patients with acute myocardial infarction. In approximately 100 patients studied in the intensive coronary care unit, serial LV ejection-fraction determinations have been obtained during the first 4 days following an acute myocardial infarction for a total of over 300 radionuclide angiograms.

During the acute phase, i.e., the first 4 days after infarction, LV ejection fractions were inversely related to infarct size as estimated from serial CPK (creatine phosphokinase) serum enzyme curve analysis.[9] In a total of 36 patients, studied within the first 24 to 48 hr (Figure 3), ejection fractions averaged 0.50 when the infarct was estimated to be smaller than 40 CPK-g-Eq, but in patients with infarcts estimated to be larger, ejection-fraction values averaged significantly lower.

A comparison was made between the noninvasive calculation of ejection fraction by the radionuclide method and LV filling pressure as determined from wedge-pressure tracings obtained by the introduction of a Swan Ganz catheter into the pulmonary artery in the wedge position. Ejection fractions averaged only 0.35 when the LV filling pressure exceeded the normal upper limit of 12 mm Hg but averaged 0.47 when the LV filling pressure was normal (Figure 4). More significantly, the majority of patients showing a serial decline in LV filling pressure toward the normal level demonstrated a corresponding increase in ejection fraction between the initial and follow-up determination. Conversely, an elevation in the LV filling pressure during the first 3–4 days was associated with

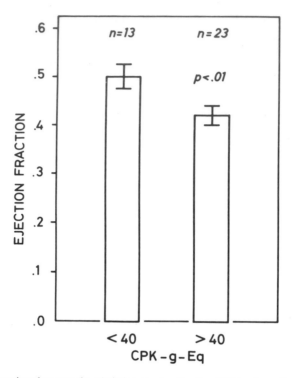

FIGURE 3. Comparison between the admission ejection fraction (EF) by the radionuclide dilution method in 36 patients with acute myocardial infarction and the estimated infarct size using the serial creatinine phosphokinase (CPK) method of Sobel *et al.*[9]

an average deterioration in left-ventricular ejection fraction as calculated by the radionuclide technique.

The serial determinations of ejection fraction have appeared to be of some prognosticative value, as judged by our intial experience. In 33 patients with an initially low or further decreasing ejection fraction in the first 4 days, there were 5 early deaths (15%), in contrast to no deaths within the first 30 days following infarction among 18 patients in whom ejection fractions were initially normal or in whom values improved during the first 4 days.

Some logistical as well as financial considerations ensue from the necessity of transporting a scintillation camera and data-recording equipment to a location, such as the coronary care unit which is required by the method we have described. With the increasing availability of excellent-quality portable scintillation cameras, which include digital magnetic tape-recording capabilities, there should be no difficulty in obtaining suitable equipment for use in various hospital locations. Simiarly, dedicated digital analytical systems are becoming more familiar to nuclear medicine specialists. Justification for the cost of such equipment may be in question if one envisions utilization of these expensive devices solely for occasional cardiac evaluation in smaller community hospitals. On the other hand, it is not difficult to imagine that this equipment might be shared between the nuclear medicine and cardiology services in order to ensure maximum utilization.

In view of recent developments in the use of single-probe systems for ejection-fraction determination, one might question the wisdom of using a scintillation camera for this purpose at all. The simplicity as well as the reduced cost of a single-probe system certainly has many advantages, particularly for smaller clinics and in those special applications in which serial estimates of various parameters of cardiac and pulmonary performance are desired. The most compelling argument, however, for a portable scintillation camera is that these now rather commonly available devices would appear to be capable of a far greater range of cardiac and pulmonary examinations, e.g., lung perfusion and ventilation imaging, myocardial scanning, acute "infarct" imaging, ECG-gated ventricular-wall-motion studies, than is possible with a single-probe system.

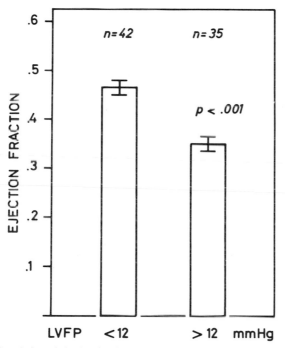

FIGURE 4. Correlation of ejection fraction (EF) and LV filling pressure (LVFP) in 77 consecutive measurements in which both determinations were made. Normal LVFP is less than 12 mm Hg.

Summary

It is our conclusion that it is possible to obtain reliable measurements of left-ventricular ejection fraction by analysis of the LV time-activity curve following the intravenous injection of a bolus of a physiologically inert substance, such as ^{99m}Tc-labeled human serum albumin. The safety and relative simplicity of the method should lend itself well to the study of LV function in acutely ill patients as well as in the serial evaluation of patients with ischemic heart disease on an outpatient basis without resorting to more invasive techniques, such as contrast angiography. In addition, since the method is primarily based on a continuous recording of count-rate fluctuations from within a fixed sampling "window" (i.e., region of interest) it would appear to depend less on an intact LV geometry as required for area-length calculations (e.g., echocardiography), which is often lacking in patients with extensive wall-motion abnormalities.

Acknowledgment

This work was supported in part by National Heart and Lung Institute Grants HL-14197 and HL-17682 and NHLI contract No. 1-HV-81332.

References

1. Weber, P. M., dos Remedios, L. V., and Jasko, I. A., Quantitative radioisotopic angiocardiography, *J. Nucl. Med.* *13:*815–822 (1972).
2. Steele, P. P., Van Dyke, D., Trow, R. S., Anger, H. O., and Davies, H., Simple and safe bedside method for serial measurement of left ventricular ejection fraction, cardiac output, and pulmonary blood volume, *Br. Heart J.* *36:*122–131 (1974).
3. Steele, P., Kirch, D., Matthews, M., and Davies, H., Measurement of left heart ejection fraction and end-diastolic volume by a computerized, scintigraphic technique using a wedged pulmonary artery catheter, *Amer. J. Cardiol.* *34:*179–186 (1974).
4. Schelbert, H. R., Verba, J. W., Johnson, A. D., Brock, G. W., Alazraki, N. P., Rose, F. J., and Ashburn, W. L., Non-traumatic determination of left ventricular ejection fraction by radionuclide angiocardiography, *Circulation* *51:*902–909 (1975).
5. Van Dyke, D., Anger, H. O., Sullivan, R. W., Vetter, W. R., Yano, Y., and Parker, H. G., Cardiac evaluation from radioisotope dynamics, *J. Nucl. Med.* *13:*585–592 (1972).
6. Mullins, C. B., Mason, D. T., Ashburn, W. L., and Ross, J., Jr., Determination of left ventricular volume by radioisotope-angiography, *Amer. J. Cardiol.* *24:*72, 78 (1969).
7. Strauss, H. W., Zaret, B. L., Hurley, P. J., Natarjan, T. K., and Pitt, B., Ascintiphotographic method for measuring left ventricular ejection fraction in man without cardiac catheterization, *Amer. J. Cardiol.* *28:*575–580 (1971).
8. Bonte, F. J., Parkey, R. W., Graham, K. D., Moore, J., and Stokely, E. M., A new method for radionuclide imaging of myocardial infarcts, *Radiology* *110:*473, 474 (1974).
9. Sobel, B. E., Bresnahan, B. F., Shell, W. E., *et al.,* Estimation of infarct size in man and its relation to prognosis, *Circulation* *46:*640–648 (1972).

Simplified Techniques for Radioangiographic Analysis

D. D. Watson, J. J. Greenberg, F. J. Hildner,
R. R. Sankey, and A. J. Gilson

Introduction

A variety of equipment is available and in use today that allows the formation of curves of activity as a function of time from selected cardiac chambers and lung fields in conjunction with the radionuclide cardiac-flow study. These radionuclide indicator–dilution (RID) curves can be analyzed to yield information about the hemodynamic status of cardiopulmonary circulation. In this study, RID curves were obtained from a scintillation camera, interfaced to a small on-line computer, and studies were performed pre- and postoperatively on patients undergoing heart surgery. The results from the preoperative studies have been compared with cardiac catheterization data which were available in every case.

Three parameters that can be quickly and easily extracted from the RID curves have been adopted for routine use. These parameters are mean central transit time (MCTT), pulmonary delay time (PDT), and left mixing time (LMT). The method of obtaining these parameters and their relation to the catheterization data will be the subject of this discussion.

D. D. WATSON, J. J. GREENBERG, R. R. SANKEY, A. J. GILSON, and F. J. HILDNER · Departments of Radiology, Thoracic Surgery, and Cardiology, Baumritter Institute of Nuclear Medicine, Mount Sinai Medical Center, Miami Beach, Florida.

Methods

Patients are placed supine beneath a scintillation camera, interfaced to the computer system. A sheet source containing ^{99m}Tc is placed beneath the patient, and the patient is positioned by viewing the cardiac silhouette on a persistence oscilloscope. A transmission image of the cardiac silhouette is then recorded. The sheet source is removed, and 10–15 mCi ^{99m}Tc pertechnetate is injected as a bolus. The injection method has been discussed in another paper.[1] In brief, a blood-pressure cuff at 40 mm Hg is used to elevate the intravenous pressure of the arm. The cuff is then raised to above systolic pressure, and the injection is made into a tributary of the basilic vein, after which the cuff is released. Serial images are recorded by the camera and the computer at the rate of 1 frame/sec. After the study, computer-generated cursors are located over the superior vena cava, right ventricle, right lung, and left ventricle. The computer then generates RID curves from the selected regions.

Data were taken from 90 preoperative studies on patients scheduled for surgery for valvular or coronary artery disease. Catheterization was usually performed a few days prior to the radionuclide study. In performing the radionuclide study, patients were maintained at rest for a few minutes prior to injection, but no other controls were exercised to ensure basal cardiac output. Disparities caused by normal short-term changes in cardiac output or by departure from basal conditions will therefore be reflected in these results.

Analysis of Data

Parameters obtained from the RID curves[2–4] are the mean central transit time (MCTT), the pulmonary delay time (PDT), and the left mixing time (LMT), as illustrated in Figure 1. The MCTT is the time interval between the centroids of the curves obtained from the right ventricle and the left ventricle. The PDT is the time interval between the centroid of the curve obtained from the right ventricle and the peak of the curve obtained from the left ventricle. The LMT is the time obtained by taking the interval from half-height to the centroid of the left ventricle curve and subtracting the half-height-to-centroid interval of the right-ventricle curve.

Proper determination of the curve centroids is essential to the analysis of RID curves. Conventional methods that require the curve tails to be separated from background and recirculation are difficult and potentially inaccurate. An alternate method that has proved accurate and reproducible has been developed for this work. The method is as follows:

For the right-ventricle (RV) curve, if C_p is the peak concentration, then the

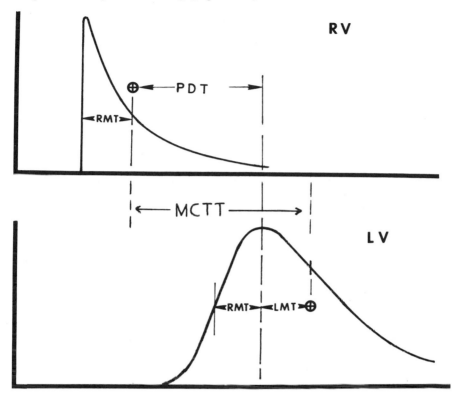

FIGURE 1. Time activity curves obtained from cursors located over the right ventricle and the left ventricle, showing the determination of MCTT, PDT, and LMT.

centroid $\bar{t}$ will be the point C_t of the downslope, where

$$C_t = \frac{1}{e}\left(1 + \frac{BT}{DT}\right)C_p$$

where BT is the build-up time (time from half-height to peak), and DT is the decay time (time from peak to half-height).

For the left-ventricle (LV) curves, the best and most consistent estimate of the true centroid is the same as for the RV curve, except that the point C_t becomes

$$C_t = \frac{2}{e}\, C_p$$

Use of this method will reveal that adequate results would ordinarily be obtained simply by locating the centroid positions at the 50% point on the downslope of the RV curve and the 75% point on the downslope of the LV curve.

Discussion of Results

The distribution of values obtained from the measurements of MCTT is shown in Figure 2. The normal value for MCTT obtained for this group, which had an average age of 56 years, was 9.0±1.2 sec. This agrees with the values 8.54±1.1 for RV to LV and 9.2±1.2 for RA to LV obtained by Jones *et al.*[5] for a group of normal subjects. From these results, greater than 11 sec will be properly classified as prolonged with 95% statistical certainty or with 99% statistical certainty for values of MCTT greater than 12 sec. Factors that cause prolonged MCTT are decreased cardiac output, valvular insufficiency, or elevated central blood volumes. Prolonged MCTT is therefore a definite indication of hemodynamic abnormality but is nonspecific of the cause. Patients with coronary artery disease or with valvular stenosis have normal MCTT unless there is concomitant valvular insufficiency, elevated atrial or ventricular volume, or reduced cardiac output.

The PDT is a measure of the average delay time of indicator passing through the pulmonary vasculature. It is proposed for use as a simple approximate indicator of reduced resting cardiac index (cardiac output normalized to total body surface area). Figure 3 shows the observed relationship between PDT and the cardiac index (CI) determined at catheterization. The solid line is the relation

$$CI = 15.6/PDT \qquad (1)$$

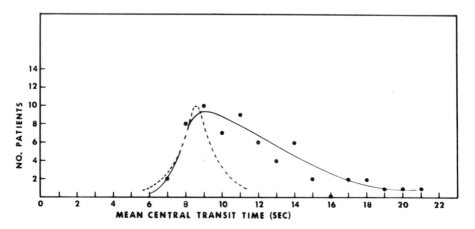

FIGURE 2. Solid line—Distribution of values obtained for patients with acquired heart disease. Dotted line—Normal distribution of 8.5±1.1 sec.

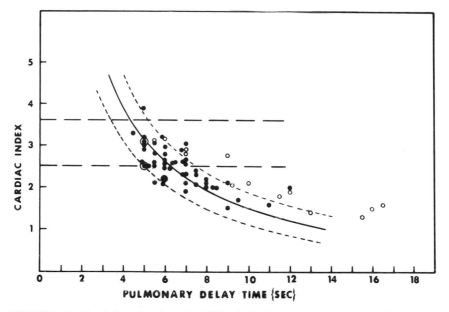

FIGURE 3. Cardiac index plotted against PDT. Solid line—Equation CI = 15.6/PDT; dotted lines—±20% variations. Normal range of CI between 2.5 and 3.5 is also indicated.

which is a simplified approximation for the cardiac index, demonstrating that CI is approximately inversely proportional to PDT. The dotted lines indicate variations of ±20%. Variations of this magnitude are typical when two methods of measuring cardiac output are compared if the measurements are not performed simultaneously. Thus, the variations shown in Figure 3 will, in part, be demonstrating typical daily variations in cardiac output or failure to achieve basal output when special preparation of the patient is not employed. The simplified relationship (Eq. 1) systematically underestimates the CI in cases of mitral incompetence or in cases of left heart failure, in which case PDT may be prolonged more than in inverse proportion to the reduction in CI. This would be caused by elevated pulmonary blood volume in these states, which is not accounted for by the simple inverse relation (Eq. 1). However, these effects do not alter the utility of PDT for the purpose of classification. Values of PDT in excess of 7.5 sec may be taken to indicate reduced resting cardiac index; values of PDT between 6.5 and 7.5 sec are equivocal. The PDT is not used to indicate CI if the sequential scintiphotos reveal an abnormal pulmonary vascular pattern or large left atrium.

The LMT is a measure of the amount of bolus spread contributed specifically by the left heart, and it is proposed for use as an indicator of abnormal rate of clearance from the left heart. Figure 4 shows the distribution of values obtained for LMT. Values from 3 to 4 sec indicate a normal rate of clearance from

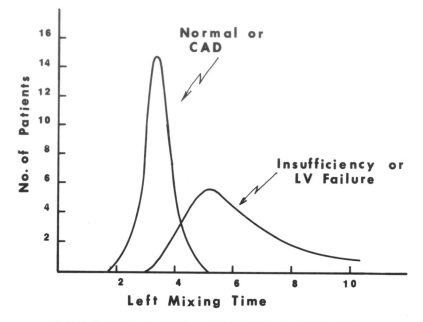

FIGURE 4. Distribution of values of LMT for the classifications indicated.

the left heart. The finding of prolonged LMT is always accompanied by the finding of "prolonged downslope" of the dye-dilution curve, obtained from pulmonary arterial injection with femoral arterial sampling at catheterization. The technique is therefore considered to be successful in separating the effects of bolus dilution and spreading contributed by the injection, right heart, and lungs from the bolus dilution that takes place in the left heart. Prolonged LMT may reflect impaired myocardial function or mitral or aortic insufficiency, but it does not differentiate between valvular or myocardial disease. In this group, two cases of well-compensated aortic insufficiency demonstrated normal LMT. All other cases of insufficiency or reduced output had prolonged LMT.

Summary

Radionuclide-indicator dilution curves have been obtained from an intravenous bolus injection of ^{99m}Tc pertechnetate. A simplified analysis of the curves was performed to obtain three parameters: MCTT, PDT, and LMT, which were compared with findings at catheterization and surgery. The MCTT provides an overall indication of central hemodynamic performance; and the PDT can serve as an indication of reduced resting cardiac index.

This method offers greater simplicity and does not require the determination of blood volume or the use of special intravascular radionuclide preparations nor does it require corrections for recirculation, background, and scattering, as are required by the conventional method of cardiac-output measurement from RID curves. The LMT demonstrated cases of prolonged clearance from the left heart regardless of variable amounts of bolus spreading prior to entering the left heart. However, the RID curves do not differentiate the cause of delayed left heart clearance. Differentiation between valvular or myocardial dysfunction can be made using the high-frequency analysis of systolic and diastolic events.

The RID parameters discussed here can be simply and rapidly obtained, and provide objective indications of hemodynamic abnormalities that cannot be obtained by visual inspection of sequential scintiphotos.

Acknowledgment

This work was supported by USPHS Grant HL-15780.

References

1. Watson, D. D., Nelson, J. P., and Gottlieb, S., Rapid bolus injection of radioisotopes, *Radiology* *106:*347–352 (February 1973).
2. Watson, D. D., Sankey, R. R., Kenny, P. J., Smoak, W. M., Yahr, Y. Z., and Gilson, A. J., *Cardiac Evaluation,* Chap. 8, Continuing education lecutures, Southeastern Chapter, Society of Nuclear Medicine (1974).
3. Watson, D. D., and Nelson, J. P., A mixing dispersion model for radiocardiographic studies (to be published).
4. Donato, L., Quantitative radiocardiography and myocardial blood flow measurements with radioisotopes, IAEA-SM-136/*208:*645–664 (1970).
5. Jones, R. H., Goodrich, J. K., and Sabiston, D. C., Quantitative radionuclide angiocardiography in evaluation of cardiac function, *Surg. Forum, 22* (1971).

Value of Combined Hemodynamic and Radiocardiographic Studies in Acute Respiratory Failure

James H. Ellis, Jr. and Peter P. Steele

Introduction

Hemodynamic abnormalities may result from or precipitate acute respiratory failure from a variety of etiologies. Thus, the clinical assessment of associated left ventricular dysfunction or pulmonary embolism may be difficult, particularly with severe underlying chronic obstructive lung disease, extensive pneumonia, or the adult respiratory-distress syndrome. In these situations rales and rhonchi are common and may obscure heart sounds. ECG abnormalities may be nonspecific, and portable chest radiographs taken in the anteroposterior view make interpretation of subtle changes in cardiac silhouette and lung parenchyma difficult.

A radioisotopic method has been recently developed for measuring cardiac and pulmonary circulatory function, and we have combined data from this technique with those from bedside right heart catheterization to study patients who are seriously ill with respiratory failure. This method provides an approach to understanding both cardiac and pulmonary physiologic abnormalities that can complicate or precipitate acute respiratory failure. This report extends the original observations of bedside radiocardiography and presents evidence that further establishes its clinical value.[1]

JAMES H. ELLIS, JR. and PETER P. STEELE·Department of Medicine, Denver Veterans Administration Hospital, University of Colorado Medical Center, Denver, Colorado.

Methods

We have studied 125 patients with acute ventilatory failure ($Pa_{O_2} <$ 50 mm Hg) of diverse etiology (chronic bronchitis and emphysema, asthma, pulmonary edema, neurological disease, radiation fibrosis, trauma, pulmonary embolism, atelectasis, and adult respiratory-distress syndrome). Of the 125 patients, 84 (67%) had an elevated Pa_{CO_2} and acute respiratory acidosis. All patients were men with a mean age of 63 yr. Twenty-eight patients had severe, well-documented, chronic obstructive lung disease as evidenced by prior pulmonary function screening within 4 years of admission (FVC 2.18±0.77 L; avg ± SD; $FEV_{1.0}$ 0.84±0.30 L; % $FEV_{1.0}$/FVC 39±11). Nineteen additional patients had historical, roentgenographic, and physical evidence of moderate to severe obstructive-airways disease. Sixty-nine (55%) of the patients required assisted or controlled mechanical ventilation, and all patients were studied in the medical or surgical intensive care units.

A method has been developed for performing radiocardiography that utilizes a portable scintillation probe (2×2 in. sodium iodide crystal), a high-frequency ratemeter, and a rapid-response strip-chart recorder along with ^{113m}In.[1] This radionuclide rapidly binds to transferrin, and thus can be used to measure blood volume and cardiac output[2] in addition to left-ventricular ejection fraction, pulmonary transit time, and pulmonary blood volume.

Study of the patient requires the insertion of a catheter into the superior or inferior vena cava for the injection of 1.0 mCi ^{113m}In with recording of its passage through the central circulation by the scintillation probe placed over the precordium in the supine anteroposterior projection. Proper collimation of the probe over the midpoint of the left ventricle is achieved by taping a radiopaque marker to the skin over the estimated midpoint of the left ventricle and then taking a portable supine anteroposterior chest film. From the roentgenogram, the position of the catheter in a central vein and the true midpoint of the left ventricle, relative to the marker, can be confirmed. Alternately, the mid-left ventricle

Editor's Note: The need for simple bedside techniques that can be applied to the critically ill patient who is often monitored in an intensive care unit because of the gravity of his cardiopulmonary condition is of the utmost importance to the practicing physician. Oftentimes in these critically ill patients, definitive data to assess their current status and response to therapy are required at short notice. The availability of recently developed, easily performed radioisotopic cardiac studies as described by the authors illustrates that these techniques can be applied at the bedside. Moreover, they can be repeated safely to assess the patient's condition or associated cardiopulmonary complications. The safe noninvasive radiocardiographic studies described by the authors have been found to be useful in this group of critically ill patients with respiratory failure.

can be marked fluoroscopically. The correct position for the probe is then marked on the chest with a felt pen to ensure accurate repositioning of the probe for serial studies.

Quantitative radiocardiography yields the following:

1. Cardiac output (CO) from area measurement of the first pass (corrected for recirculation), count rate at equilibrium (5 min), and total blood volume.
2. Pulmonary transit time (PTT); time from 75% of the right ventricular peak count rate to the left ventricular (LV) peak.
3. Pulmonary blood volume (PBV); product of PTT and CO. Cardiac index and PBV index can be determined from the estimated body surface area by division.
4. Left-ventricular ejection fraction (LVEF); the ratio of the peak (LV end-diastolic count rate) to the valley (LV end-systolic count rate) and the ratio of the end-diastolic peak to the corresponding point on the eclipse record (see Figure 1). For calculation of LVEF, radiation scatter is empirically corrected by recording a second time-activity curve at one-half the initial [113m]In dose with the LV eclipsed such that activity is recorded from the tissues surrounding the LV. That curve is presented as the solid line beneath the upper curve, which is drawn by matching the trailing edges of the two records (see Figure 1).

These four aspects of central circulatory function as determined with [113m]In and the scintillation probe have been validated with standard techniques.[1-4] Thus, total blood volume measured with [113m]In compared favorably with blood volume measured with ^{125}I-serum albumin ($r = 0.80; P < 0.001; n = 9$). CO measured with the scintillation probe and [113m]In correlated with CO measured with indocyanine-green dye (Stewart-Hamilton) ($r = 0.78; P < 0.001; n = 35$). PTT and PBV determined in dogs,[3,4] using the radionuclide technique, compared well with these measurements made with indocyanine-green dye ($r = 0.90, n = 96$ and $r = 0.80, n = 96$, respectively; $P < 0.001$). LVEF measured with the scintillation probe correlated with this measurement made with cine left ventriculography (area length, single plane) ($r = 0.90; P < 0.001; n = 67$).

Bedside right heart catheterization, using the Swan-Ganz catheter,[5] was performed in 64 of these patients. Vascular pressures were monitored with P23Ia Statham transducers positioned 5 cm below the angle of Louis in the supine patient and recorded on an Electronics for Medicine IR-4C Recorder, which also monitored and recorded the ECG. Of 71 catheterizations attempted, 64 (90%) were successful in that the pulmonary artery could be catheterized and the pulmonary-artery wedge pressure could be obtained. There were no complications from these procedures, the frequency of premature beats was minimal, and only the complete, successful catheterization data are herein reported.

Results

Patients with acute respiratory failure could be categorized into one of four groups according to the radiocardiographic pattern: (1) Normal; (2) short pulmonary transit time (short PTT); (3) right ventricular dysfunction (RVD); (4) left ventricular dysfunction (LVD). The four patterns are illustrated in Figure 1.

Although pattern recognition is in itself often sufficient for clinical management, the value of quantitation of central circulatory dynamics, using bedside radiocardiography and right heart catheterization, are presented in this report. The results of evaluation of 125 patients with acute respiratory failure are presented in Table 1.

1. Normal Pattern. This pattern was noted in the greatest number of cases (50 of 125; 40%). Mean cardiac index (CI), PBV index, and LVEF were within normal limits (Table 1). An example of a normal radiocardiographic pattern is shown in Figure 2, and it is representative of the radiocardiograms found in this group of patients. The PBV index of 343 ± 97 ml/m² is in agreement with other published data for estimating PBV.[6]

Right heart catheterization was performed in 20 patients with a normal radiocardiogram. Elevation of mean pulmonary artery (PA) pressure was noted in all patients, and a correlation between the mean right atrial (RA) and the mean pulmonary-artery wedge (PAW) pressures is observed ($r = 0.68$) (Figure 3). Although most patients with a normal LVEF had a normal mean PAW pressure, 3 had elevation of PAW to greater than 15 mm Hg with concomitant elevation of RA pressure. The cause of this abnormal elevation in right- and left-ventricular filling pressures is uncertain, but could represent transmission of increased intrapleural pressure. There was no clinical evidence of left ventricular hypertrophy in these patients, but altered ventricular compliance could be present.

Fifteen of these 50 patients (30%) died as a result of progressive respiratory insufficiency, sepsis, gastrointestinal hemorrhage, or cerebral vascular accident. None died of cardiac failure. Autopsies were performed in 13 of the 15 patients who died, and there was no evidence of pulmonary emboli or significant coronary artery disease (CAD). RV hypertrophy (RV wall thickness $\geqslant$ 5 mm) was noted in 5 patients, and severe chronic bronchitis and emphysema was present at autopsy in each case. CAD was absent or mild (as defined as less than 20% occlusion of any major vessel) in all patients. Thus, a normal precordial radiocardiogram suggests the absence of major pulmonary thromboembolism and normal cardiac performance.

2. Short Pulmonary Transit-Time Pattern. The short PTT pattern is characterized by loss of the distinct separation of right and left-ventricular peaks with very rapid arrival of the isotope to the left side of the heart, as shown in Figure 4.

This pattern was noted in 23 patients (18%). If the left-ventricular peak cannot be distinguished with certainty, injection of ^{113m}In into the main PA will

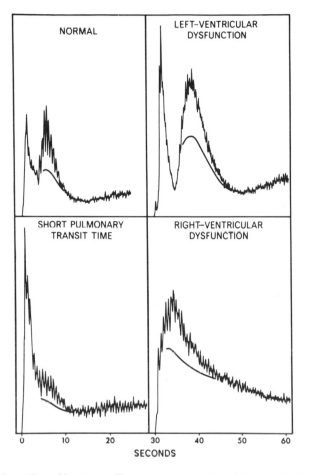

FIGURE 1. Radiocardiographic patterns. The normal radiocardiographic pattern is characterized by a normal or increased cardiac index with distinct right- and left-ventricular peaks. Pulmonary blood volume (PBV) is normal and left-ventricular ejection fraction (LVEF) is ≥55%. The left-ventricular dysfunction (LVD) pattern is characterized by a decrease in LVEF to <.55%. The short pulmonary transit time (PTT) pattern is characterized by lack of distinct separation of right and left heart peaks, usually a normal cardiac index, and a marked decrease in PBV. The right-ventricular dysfunction (RVD) pattern is characterized by slow washout of the radionuclide from the right heart with subsequent loss of distinct right and left heart peaks, but PBV is normal or increased.

**TABLE 1. Results of Radiocardiographic and Hemodynamic Studies
in Acute Respiratory Failure**

	Radiographic pattern			
	Normal	Short PTT	RVD	LVD
Patients	50 (40%)	23 (18%)	21 (17%)	31 (25%)
Cardiac index				
(L/min/m²)	3.31 ± 1.11	3.18 ± 1.24	2.90 ± 1.01	2.42 ± 1.00
Pulmonary blood				
volume index,				
(ml/m²)	343 ± 97	186 ± 70	391 ± 89	382 ± 113
Left ventricular				
ejection fraction (%)	67 ± 9	63 ± 6	62 ± 7	32 ± 13
Right-heart				
catheterization,				
pressures (mm Hg)[b]	n^a = 20	n = 12	n = 15	n = 17
RA	9 ± 4	8 ± 4	14 ± 8	8 ± 4
PA	32 ± 13	33 ± 9	43 ± 11	44 ± 13
PAW	11 ± 4	9 ± 5	14 ± 7	17 ± 10
Deaths	15 (30%)	11 (48%)	8 (38%)	18 (58%)

[a]n = number of procedures.
[b]Pressures, mean mm Hg; (RA) right atrium; (PA) pulmonary artery; (PAW) pulmonary artery wedge; mean ±
SD.

establish the PTT (Figure 4). The decrease in PBV index (186 ± 70 ml/m²) in these patients is significantly different from normal ($P < 0.01$) (Table 1). It is important to realize that since PBV is the product of CO and PTT, with a marked reduction in CO, PBV can be reduced with a normal PTT.

Right heart catheterization in 12 patients with a short PTT pattern revealed an elevated mean PA pressure to a level not different from those patients with a normal pattern (Table 1). RA and PAW pressures appear to correlate well (Figure 5).

Eleven of 23 patients (48%) died, and autopsy examination was performed in 10 of these cases. All 10 had multiple or massive pulmonary emboli and normal left ventricles. Perfusion lung scans were abnormal when performed in 17 of 23 patients. Thus, the radiocardiogram defines a group of patients with ventilatory failure who have marked reduction in pulmonary blood volume, and correlation with major pulmonary embolism seems established.

3. Right-Ventricular Dysfunction Pattern. The RVD pattern is characterized by a complete or partial loss of distinct right and left ventricular peaks, similar, at first, to that due to a short PTT pattern but with a normal PBV. Figure 6 presents a radiocardiographic tracing in a patient with severe chronic obstructive-airways disease and cor pulmonale. It is evident that the LV peak cannot be accurately localized in this particular case, and for clarification of

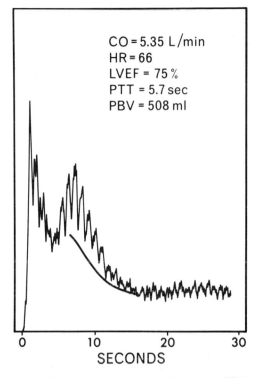

CO = 5.35 L/min
HR = 66
LVEF = 75 %
PTT = 5.7 sec
PBV = 508 ml

SECONDS

FIGURE 2. Normal radiocardiographic pattern. (CO) cardiac output; (HR) heart rate; (LVEF) left-ventricular ejection fraction; (PTT) pulmonary transit time; (PBV) pulmonary blood volume. See the text for methods of measurement.

pulmonary transit time, necessary for calculation of PBV, pulmonary artery catheterization for delivery of the radionuclide is frequently essential. Twenty-one patients (17%) demonstrated the RVD pattern, and all the patients in this series had severe, far-advanced, obstructive-airways disease that was evident clinically and confirmed by autopsy.

Right heart catheterization was performed in 15 patients, and a marked elevation of mean PA pressure (43 ± 11 mm Hg) is striking and significantly elevated over a mean PA pressure noted in patients with the normal radiocardiogram ($P <. 0.05$) (Table 1). There is good correlation between the mean RA and PAW pressures ($r = 0.94$) (Figure 7).

Seven of the 15 had an elevation of PAW to more than 15 mm Hg in association with a normal LVEF, which probably reflects the fluid retention due to right heart failure and not LV failure.

Eight of 20 (38%) patients with the RVD pattern died, which was not different from the patients with a normal radiocardiogram, and autopsies were

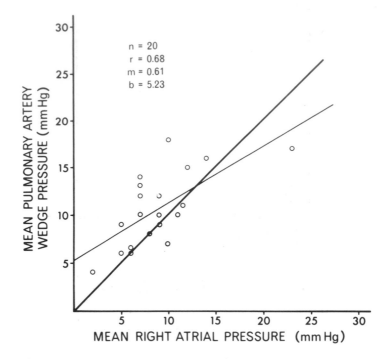

FIGURE 3. Correlation between mean right atrial and pulmonary artery wedge pressures in 20 patients with a normal radiocardiogram. (*r*) Correlation coefficient; (*m*) slope; (*b*) intercept. The fine line represents the line of best fit; the heavy line represents the line of identity.

performed in 4 patients. Examination showed that their left ventricles were normal, and there was no evidence of coronary artery disease. Also, none had pulmonary emboli. The striking abnormality was marked RV dilatation with minimal hypertrophy (the greatest RV wall thickness was 5 mm in one patient). Thus, a radiocardiogram with indistinct right and left heart peaks suggest either right ventricular dysfunction or major pulmonary embolism. Loss of the distinct separation due to RVD must be distinguished from that due to reduction in pulmonary blood volume. In most patients, the PA injection is necessary to determine PTT and PBV, as in the unusual case with markedly decreased cardiac output.

4. Left-Ventricular Dysfunction Pattern. This pattern is defined as a decrease in LVEF to < 55%. Thirty-one (25%) patients demonstrated this pattern with a mean LVEF of 32±13%. An example of this radiocardiographic pattern is presented in Figure 8.

In this particular patient and the majority of cases, the RV peak and pulmo-

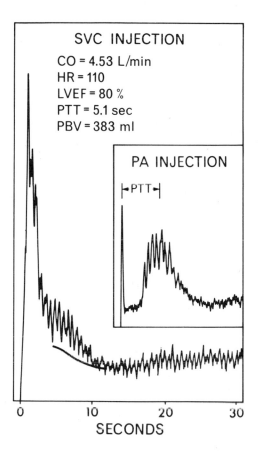

FIGURE 1. Short pulmonary transit time (PTT) pattern. The superior vena caval (SVC) injection demonstrates the typical pattern of rapid labeling of the left ventricle, but a pulmonary artery (PA) injection may be necessary to accurately measure pulmonary transit time (PTT) and consequently pulmonary blood volume (PBV). (Abbreviations as in Figure 2.)

nary valley are clearly distinguished, and PTT and PBV can be calculated. However, in some patients the LV dilatation is so marked that the RV peak cannot be seen on the LV collimated tracing, and PTT and PBV are determined from the combination of the LV collimated and eclipse tracings (Figure 9).

The lowest LVEF that is calculable from the radiocardiographic pattern is 20%, since this appears as oscillations that are indistinguishable from the background radiation or "noise."

Right heart catheterization was performed in 17 patients with LV dysfunc-

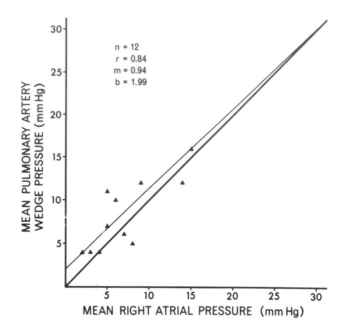

FIGURE 5. Correlation between RA and PAW pressures in a short PTT pattern. (Symbols as in Figure 3.)

tion, and the mean PA pressure (44±13 mm Hg) was significantly elevated over the pressures seen in the normal pattern ($P < 0.05$) (Table 1). Of interest is the correlation between the mean RA and PAW pressures, as shown in Figure 10, with marked differences between the left- and the right-ventricular filling pressures. Nine patients had a mean PAW pressure of less than 15 mm Hg in association with a reduction of LVEF.

In the LVD pattern group of patients, a subgroup with reduction of LVEF to less than 40% and a high mortality (73%) can be identified. The overall mortality of the LVD group was 58%. Autopsies were performed in 14 of the 18 who died, and all had severe coronary artery disease (greater than 80% occlusion of one or more major vessels) with old or recent myocardial infarction noted in 10. Thus, marked reduction of LVEF in acute ventilatory failure is usually associated with coronary artery disease and a poor prognosis.

The relationship between LVEF and mean PAW pressure is shown in Figure 11. For patients with a normal radiocardiogram, 17 of 20 (85%) had a PAW pressure of 15 mm Hg or less over an LVEF range of 55%–80%. Patients with RVD pattern had variable PAW pressures with 8 of 14 (57%) having elevated PAW pressures. Eight of 17 (47%) patients with LVD pattern had elevated PAW

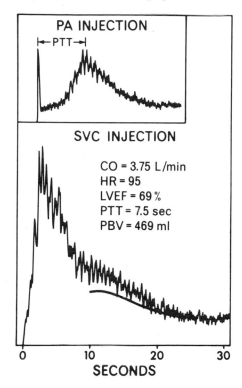

FIGURE 6. Right-ventricular dysfunction (RVD) pattern. Note that in the superior vena caval (SVC) injection tracing, the PTT cannot be determined. The pulmonary artery (PA) injection tracing represents injection of ¹¹³ᵐIn into the main PA, thus bypassing interference from the right ventricle so that PTT can be determined. (Abbreviations as in Figure 2.)

pressures. The case and safety of bedside right heart catheterization with the flow-directed Swan-Ganz catheter, and the poor correlation ($r = 0.44$) of mean PAW pressure with LVEF, suggest that these measurements complement rather than compete with one another in the management of the seriously ill patient with acute respiratory failure.

Discussion

Precordial radiocardiography and bedside right heart catheterization with the Swan Ganz catheter can be easily and safely applied to the seriously ill patient with acute ventilatory failure. We record the radiocardiogram first and decide on the desirability of right heart catheterization based on the radiocardiogram. Based on our data, we utilize right heart catheterization when there is a reduction of LVEF or when low cardiac output is present with a normal LVEF.

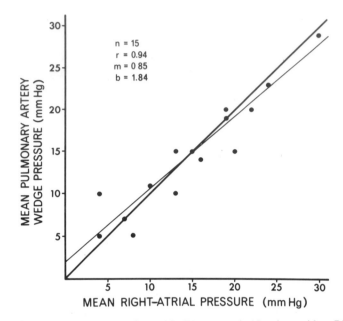

FIGURE 7. Correlation between mean RA and PAW pressures in 15 patients with an RVD pattern. (Symbols as in Figure 3.)

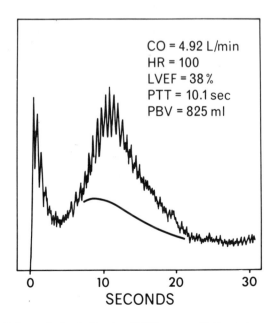

FIGURE 8. Left-ventricular dysfunction (LVD) pattern. (Abbreviations as in Figure 2.)

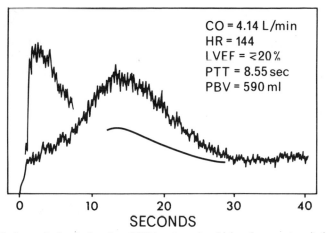

FIGURE 9. Left-ventricular dysfunction (LVD) pattern, in which pulmonary transit time is determined by a combination of collimated and eclipsed tracings.

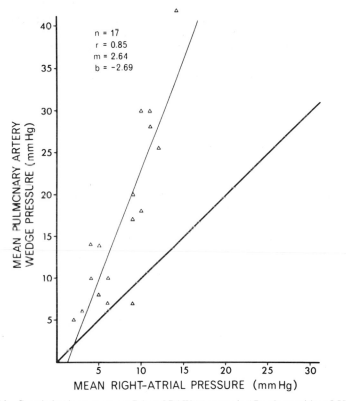

FIGURE 10. Correlation between mean RA and PAW pressures in 17 patients with an LVD pattern. (Symbols as in Figure 3.)

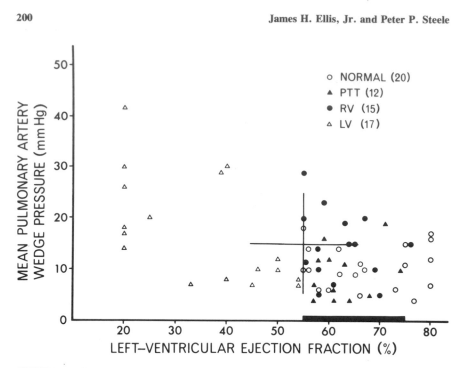

FIGURE 11. Correlation of mean pulmonary wedge pressure with left-ventricular ejection fraction in acute respiratory failure.

The clinical value of radiocardiography is reflected in the frequency (18%) of major pulmonary embolism as defined by reduced pulmonary blood volume and the frequency (25%) of impaired LVEF in acute ventilatory failure. In addition, a subgroup of patients with marked impairment of LVEF to ≲ 40%, coronary artery disease, and high mortality can be identified. With LV failure, knowledge of the LV filling pressure is advantageous.

Massive pulmonary emboli were present in all 10 patients autopsied with the short PTT pattern. Consequently there was a marked decrease in calculated PBV. Markedly abnormal perfusion defects by lung scanning were noted in all 17 of the 23 patients able to be studied in this group, but all patients had confirmed pulmonary thromboembolism. The defects were not subtle and accounted for an estimated 25–60% decrease in the area of perfused lung tissue. An average decrease of 46% in PBV index is noted when the mean PBV index in the PTT group is compared to the PBV index in the normal group. The short PTT pattern and decrease in PBV was seen only secondary to massive pulmonary embolism in this group of patients.

Quantitative bedside radiocardiography identifies cardiac and pulmonary circulatory abnormalities in acute respiratory failure.

Acknowledgment

This work was supported by Veterans Administration Research Funds, and a grant from the American Lung Association of Colorado.

References

1. Steele, P. P., Van Dyke, D., Trow, R. S., Anger, H. O., and Davies, H., A simple and safe bedside method for serial measurement of left-ventricular ejection fraction, cardiac output, and pulmonary blood volume, *Br. Heart J. 38:*122–131 (1974).
2. Hosain, P., Hosain, F., Igbal, Q. M., Carulli, N., and Wagner, H. N., Measurement of plasma volume using ^{99}Tc and ^{113m}In labelled proteins, *Br. J. Radiol. 42:*627–630 (1969).
3. Ellis, J. H., and Steele, P. P., Comparison of pulmonary blood volume determination in dogs by radiocardiographic and dye-dilution techniques (Abstract), *Clin. Res. 22:*200A (1974).
4. Ellis, J. H., and Steele, P. P., Comparison of pulmonary blood volume in dogs by radiocardiography and dye-dilution, *J Appl. Physiol. 37:*570–574 (1974).
5. Swan, H. J. C., Ganz, W., Forrester, J., Marcus, H., Diamond, G., and Chonette, D., Catheterization of the heart in man with the use of a flow-directed balloon-tipped catheter, *N. Engl. J. Med. 283:*447–451 (1970).
6. Giuntini, C., Lewis, M. L., SalesLuis, A., and Harvey, R. M., A study of pulmonary blood volume in man by quantitative radiocardiography, *J. Clin. Invest. 42:*1589–1605 (1963).

The Use of $C^{15}O_2$ in the Evaluation of Cardiac Abnormalities

Peter J. Kenny, Denny D. Watson, Warren R. Janowitz, and Albert J. Gilson

Introduction

Carbon dioxide labeled with oxygen-15 ($t_{1/2}$ = 124 sec) is a uniquely useful tracer for cardiopulmonary studies because it can be introduced selectively into the left heart by the simple noninvasive process of inhalation and breath-holding. Externally placed scintillation counters coupled with a high-speed multichannel recorder can be used to measure the rate of clearance of the tracer from the lungs and the rate of filling and emptying of the left heart. The presence of left-to-right intracardiac shunts or mitral or aortic valvular lesions can be inferred from the count rate vs. time curves. Scintigraphic images of the left ventricle in systole and diastole may be made using standard commercially available scintillation camera systems.

Our initial experience with this tracer and results of studies of normal subjects and patients with acquired heart disease are described.

Physiology

The diffusing capacity of the alveolar membrane for carbon dioxide is approximately twenty times greater than that for oxygen or carbon monoxide.[1-3]

PETER J. KENNY, DENNY D. WATSON, WARREN R. JANOWITZ, and ALBERT J. GILSON · Department of Radiology, Baumritter Institute of Nuclear Medicine, Mount Sinai Medical Center, Miami Beach, Florida.

Inhaled $C^{15}O_2$ passes rapidly through the alveolar membrane and exchanges the ^{15}O label with water in the pulmonary capillary blood according to the reaction

$$CO_2* + H_2O \rightleftharpoons H_2CO_3* \rightleftharpoons CO_2 + H_2O*$$

This reaction, which occurs within the red cell, is accelerated by the enzyme carbonic anhydrase and is complete in a small fraction of a second.[3-5] The tracer, now in the form of $H_2^{15}O$, is carried by the pulmonary venous blood into the left heart. Subsequently, during systemic circulation it rapidly equilibrates with total body water. In a healthy adult, one-half the activity is cleared from the lungs in a period of 2–5 sec. Delayed lung clearance has been observed in the presence of pulmonary edema.[6] Delayed lung clearance has also been observed in patients who were candidates for cardiac surgery for coronary artery disease or for mitral or aortic valvular lesions.[7]

Production and Administration

Oxygen-15, a 2-min half-life positron emitter, may be produced in an accelerator by bombarding ^{14}N with deuterons in the reaction ^{14}N (*d, n*) ^{15}O, or by bombarding oxygen-16 with protons in the reaction ^{16}O (*p, pn*) ^{15}O. In this work, both reactions have been employed using 26-MeV protons or 13-MeV deuterons from a medical cyclotron. The deuteron reaction is preferable since it yields carrier-free ^{15}O. Deuteron energies of 4 MeV or higher are suitable for this method of production. The ^{15}O is converted to $C^{15}O_2$ by passing the gas through an activated charcoal furnace at 550°C followed by a cupric oxide furnace at 500°C to remove traces of carbon monoxide.[8] The gas is piped directly to the clinical area, a distance of approximately 200 ft.

The patient lies in the supine position and breathes through a spirometer (with a nose clip in place). The labeled CO_2 is rapidly introduced into the mouthpiece of the spirometer tube from a 10-ml syringe while the patient is at end tidal volume. The gas abruptly enters the lungs as the patient inspires a single tidal volume and breath-holds for approximately 10 sec to ensure that all the activity diffuses completely from the alveolar space into the pulmonary capillary blood.[4] This procedure is altered when the gas is administered to an infant, in which case a nasal canula is used to introduce the labeled CO_2. The dosage normally used for cardiac function studies or left-to-right intracardiac-shunt detection is 60 Ci/kg.

Measurement

Two collimated scintillation probes, connected via single-channel spectrometers to a high-speed multichannel recorder, are used to measure the variation of activity as a function of time over the left heart and right lung as indicated schematically in Figure 1. The probes have NaI (T1) crystals $1\frac{1}{2}$ in. diameter by 1 in. thick. The spectrometers are capable of handling input count rates up to 10^5/sec without significant losses due to deadtime. Ratemeter time constants are 0.06 and 0.30 sec for the heart and lung probes, respectively; maximum observed count rates are approximately 3×10^4/sec. EKG and spirometer tracings are recorded simultaneously.

Representative Studies

The results of a typical study on a normal patient are shown in Figure 2. The beginning of inspiration, taken as zero on the time scale, is indicated by the rapid rise in count rate of the lung probe. This is followed by an exponential washout with a half-time of approximately 3.5 sec during the breath-holding period, which is indicated by the spirometer trace. There is no indication of recirculation of the tracer into the lung during this period of measurement—approximately 14 sec following inhalation. The variations of count rate shown by the heart-probe trace correspond to the filling and emptying of the left heart during the diastolic and systolic phases of the cardiac cycle. In a normal subject, it can be seen that after approximately 8 cardiac cycles, essentially all the activity has cleared the left heart.

Figure 3 shows a comparison of the principal features of the $C^{15}O_2$ curve and those of the mitral and aortic echocardiogram on the same patient. The rapidly rising portion of the $C^{15}O_2$ corresponds to early diastolic filling and follows the E wave of the anterior mitral leaflet echo. The $C^{15}O_2$ curve then levels off and is followed by a smaller filling phase corresponding in time and amplitude to the A wave of the mitral leaflet. This is presumed to be caused by

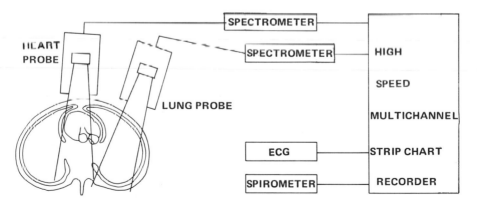

FIGURE 1. Schematic arrangement of instrumentation used to record activity vs. time curves over left heart and right lung during $C^{15}O_2$ inhalation studies.

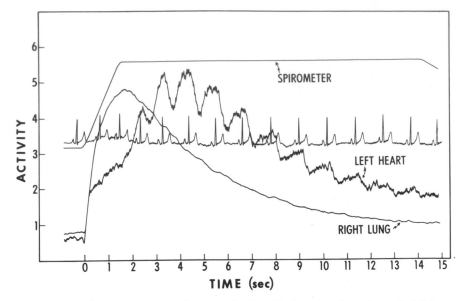

FIGURE 2. Activity vs. time curves for a normal subject. Probes are positioned over the left heart and the right lung field, as indicated in Figure 1.

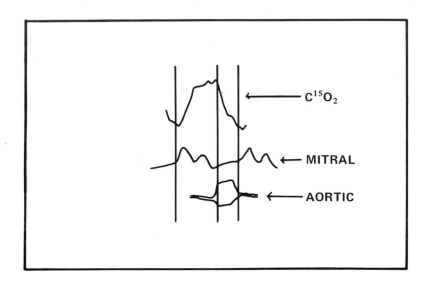

FIGURE 3. Comparison of $C^{15}O_2$ activity vs. time curve from a scintillation probe over the left ventricle with mitral and aortic echocardiograms on the same patient. The vertical lines indicate the beginning and end of the cardiac cycle with reference to the opening and closing of the aortic valve.

additional ventricular filling from atrial systole. The ventricular ejection segment begins when the aortic valve is fully open and ends when the valve is fully closed as indicated by the echo.

It is possible to calculate the total ejection fraction (TEF) from the C^{15}O$_2$ curve by taking the ratio $(D - S)/(D - B)$, where D and S are the curve amplitudes above the baseline at end-diastole, and end-systole, respectively, and B is the background contribution from all regions outside the left ventricle. The principal difficulty in making this calculation is the determination of B, which may arise from areas in the lung, left atrium, coronary arteries, and aorta, which may be partly included in the detector field of view. We have used the empirical formula

$$\text{TEF} = \frac{D - S}{D - kS}$$

where $k = 0.85$, which gives consistent results in normal subjects.[9]

The forward ejection fraction (FEF) may be calculated by plotting the amplitudes (diastolic minus systolic ordinate values) of the successive downstroke segments of the C^{15}O$_2$ heart curve as a function of time as shown in Figure 4. The FEF is then calculated from the relation

$$\text{FEF} = \frac{\text{net forward stroke volume}}{\text{end-diastolic volume}} = 2\left[1 - \exp\left(-\frac{2}{\lambda}\right)\right]$$

where λ is the number of heartbeats between the appearance time and the centroid of the curve. This formula is derived from a mathematical analysis of a two-chamber model that yields a curve of the gamma-variate form $C_t = C_0 t e^{-\lambda t}$, where C_0 and C_t are the concentrations of the tracer in the left ventricle initially and at t.

Regurgitant flow through either the mitral or aortic valve can be qualitatively recognized from a prolonged overall clearance from the heart without a concomitant reduction in ejection fraction as illustrated by Figure 5. The amount of regurgitant flow can be calculated making use of the independent measurements of forward and total ejection fraction (FEF and TEF). The left-ventricular regurgitant fraction (RF) is defined as

$$\text{RF} = \frac{\text{total stroke volume - forward stroke volume}}{\text{total stroke volume}}$$

which can be expressed as

$$\text{RF} = \frac{\text{TEF - FEF}}{\text{TEF}}$$

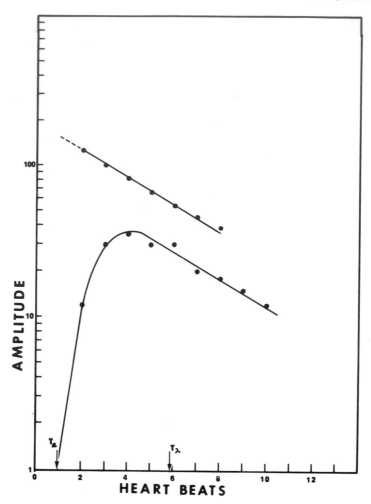

FIGURE 4. Curve resulting from plot of "down-stroke" amplitudes vs. the number of heart beats for the normal heart curve shown in Figure 2. Forward ejection fraction is calculated from this curve as described in text. The appearance time T_A and centroid T_L are indicated. The upper curve is a plot of the lung clearance rate.

Table 1 shows a comparison of TEF, FEF, AND RF on 10 normal volunteers determined by the $C^{15}O_2$ inhalation technique. As would be expected, in the absence of regurgitant flow the TEF and FEF values are equal, within the precision of the method.

Also included in Table 1 is a comparison of values determined by $C^{15}O_2$ inhalation and by catheterization on 13 cardiac patients. Reasonable agreement between the two methods is indicated.

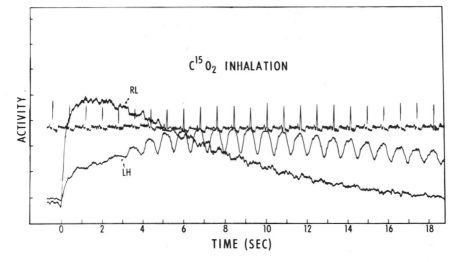

FIGURE 5. Activity vs. time curves obtained from a patient with severe aortic insufficiency show-ing qualitatively very slow overall clearance from the left heart but with a normal total systolic ejection. Quantitatively, the TEF is 72% but with an FEF of only 27% yielding an estimated regurgitant fraction of 63%.

Imaging

It is possible to obtain images of the left side of the heart following inhala-tion of $C^{15}O_2$. The absence of activity in the right heart facilitates clearer delinea-tion of the left ventricular border, and because of the penetrating 511-KeV photon from ^{15}O, the procedure yields images that are less vulnerable to absorption artifacts than those obtained with ^{99m}Tc.

A standard, commercially available imaging system (Picker Dyna-4 Camera and Gamma-11 Computer) was used. Two 2.5-in.-thick medium-energy col-limators with 1900 hexagonal holes were stacked together with the holes aligned. This arrangement provides more than adequate collimation for the 511-keV photons from ^{15}O. A 20% energy window was used, centered at 511 keV.

For the first study, a normal volunteer was used. Serial anterior images were obtained at a rate of 5/sec for 10 sec following inhalation of 40 mCi of $C^{15}O_2$. The images were stored digitally on a disk in a 64×64 matrix.

Image processing was performed as follows: A region of interest was selected encompassing the ventricle, which begins to appear approximately 2 sec following inhalation, and a count vs. time histogram was generated for this region, as shown in Figure 6, where the time units are 0.2 sec, the time for a single frame. The frames that correspond approximately to end systole and end diastole will contain the lowest and highest counts, respectively, and can be

TABLE 1. Comparative Values for Total Ejection Fraction (TEF),
Forward Ejection Fraction (FEF), and Regurgitant Fraction (RF) for Normal Subjects,
and Cardiac Patients Also Evaluated by Catheterization

	TEF		FEF	RF		
Patient	$C^{15}O_2$	Cath.	$C^{15}O_2$	$C^{15}O_2$	Catheterization	Final diagnosis[a]
A	75					Normal volunteer
B	68		64			Normal volunteer
C	73		72			Normal volunteer
D	68		64			Normal volunteer
E	69		69			Normal volunteer
F	70		64			Normal volunteer
G	71		64			Normal volunteer
H	68		72			Normal volunteer
I	70		65			Normal volunteer
J	72		71			Normal volunteer
GF	51	51	46	10[b]	0	ASHD
LK	64	69	60	6[b]	0	Normal volunteer
RH	67	78	33	50	4+regurg[c]	MI
EK	80	70	39	50	4+regurg[c]	AI
MP	79	76	76	4[b]	0	ASHD
GZ	48	47	25	48	57%	MS, AI
DS	44	46	47	0	0	ASHD
GK	60	48	51	15[b]	0	ASHD
HD	69	62	34	51	61%	MR
JA	70	64	24	66	75%	AI
RC	20	15	18		0	ASHD
DB	63	66	61	2[b]	0	ASHD
JB	80		20	75		AI (leaking prosthetic valve)

[a](AI) aortic insufficiency; (ASHD) arteriosclerotic heart disease; (MI) mitral insufficiency; (MS) mitral stenosis; (MR) mitral regurgitation.
[b]Values less than 20% considered normal.
[c]RF not calculated; *regurg* qualitatively estimated from cineangiograms.

selected from the histogram. Nine systolic and nine diastolic frames selected in this way are indicated in Figure 6.

The two sets of frames identified in Figure 6 were summed and displayed, as shown in Figure 7. A single nine-point smoothing and a 40% background subtraction has been applied to both images.

A second study was performed on an adult male volunteer with a documented history of ideopathic hypertrophic subaortic stenosis (IHSS). The same procedure was used except that the images were taken in the left anterior oblique position. Figure 8 shows the processed images corresponding to systole and diastole and the images taken at cineangiography. The position and extent of the hypertrophic lesion is clearly visualized.

A third study was performed on a patient with a documented sinus venosus atrial septal defect with a pulmonary-to-systemic-flow ratio of 3:1. Figure 9

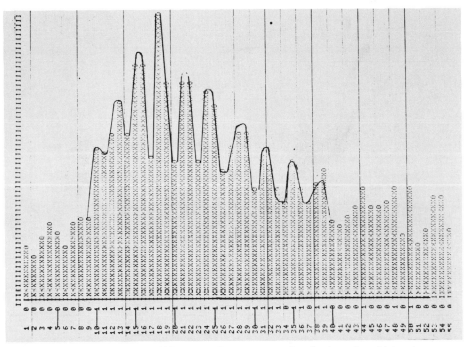

FIGURE 6. Computer-generated histogram of count rate vs. time for the region of interest encompassing the left ventricle, following inhalation of 40 mCi of $C^{15}O_2$. Time units are 0.2 sec. Peaks and valleys correspond to diastolic and systolic phases of cardiac cycle, respectively, and corresponding frames are summed to form the diastolic and systolic images. Maximum count rate is approximately 4500 cps in region of interest.

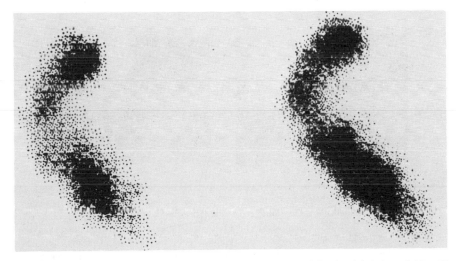

FIGURE 7. Systolic and diastolic images of a normal left heart following inhalation of 40 mCi $C^{15}O_2$. Nine-point smoothing and 40% background subtraction have been applied.

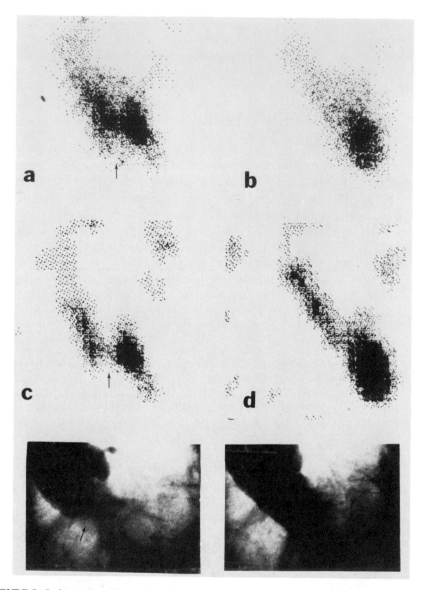

FIGURE 8. Left anterior oblique views of a patient with documented ideopathic hypertrophic sub-aortic stenosis following inhalation of 40 mCi $C^{15}O_2$. (a, b) Systolic and diastolic phase pictures. The total number of counts in the diastolic image is 8000. Position of stenotic lesion is indicated on the systolic picture. (c, d) Effect of applying a modified second spatial derivative filter to (a) and (b) to delineate the edges only. Prints were made from Tektronix 4601 hard copy unit. Cineangio pictures in systole and diastole are shown below. Position of stenotic lesion is indicated on the systolic picture.

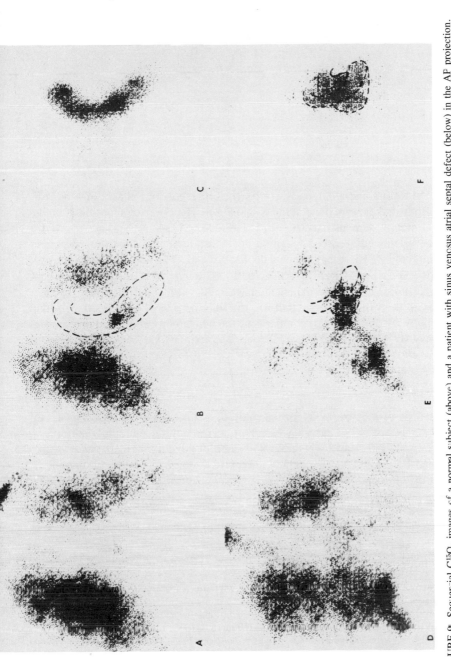

FIGURE 9. Sequential $C^{15}O_2$ images of a normal subject (above) and a patient with sinus venosus atrial septal defect (below) in the AP projection. Pulmonary-to-systemic-flow ratio in ASD is 3:1. (A) Lung phase at time of inhalation. (B) Early left atrial filling phase at 1 sec postinhalation. (C) Left heart phase. Note absence of activity in right heart. (D) Lung phase. (E) Early left-atrial filling phase showing simultaneous appearance of activity in pulmonary veins, right atrium, and left atrium, with activity appearing in the right ventricle prior to left ventricular filling. (F) Left heart phase with activity now filling all heart chambers because of shunt flow.

TABLE 2. Absorbed Radiation Dose
Following Single-Breath Inhalation
of $C^{15}O_2$

Site	mrad/mCi
Lung	5.0
Whole body	1.6
Testes	1.8
Ovaries	1.7

shows the results and a comparison with the corresponding phases of a normal study. Both studies were done in the AP position. The effect of shunt flow on the image is clearly demonstrated.

The calculated absorbed radiation doses resulting from this procedure are listed in Table 2. These have been calculated for a 70-kg adult according to the methods and data in MIRD Pamphlet No. 11. The inhaled activity is assumed to leave the lungs as a single exponential washout with a half-time of 5 sec. In addition to this, instantaneous uniform distribution and 100% retention in the whole body are assumed. For comparison, the whole body and blood doses from intravenously administered ^{99m}Tc HSA are approximately 15 and 50 mrad/mCi, respectively.

Summary

The use of inhaled $C^{15}O_2$ for the study of acquired heart disease appears to have a number of unique advantages. The tracer is introduced rapidly and selectively into the left heart by a safe, totally noninvasive method. Because of the short half-life of ^{15}O and the rapid intravascular–extravascular equilibration of the diffusible tracer, the test may be repeated within a few minutes with no interference from previously administered activity. The radiation dose is minimal, and sterility and nonpyrogenicity of the tracer do not have to be established. Finally, the test may be administered on an outpatient basis easily and rapidly.

References

1. Guyton, A. C. *Textbook of Medical Physiology,* 4th Ed., pp. 479, 480, W. B. Saunders Co., Philadelphia (1971).
2. West, J. B., Holland, R. A. B., Dollery, C. T., *et al.,* Interpretation of radioactive gas clearance rates in the lung, *J. Appl. Physiol. 17:*4–26 (1962).
3. West, J. B., *Respiratory Physiology, The Essentials,* pp. 23–32, Williams and Wilkins, Baltimore (1974).
4. West, J. B., and Dollery, C. T., Uptake of oxygen-15 labeled CO_2 compared with carbon-11 labeled CO_2 in the lung, *J. Appl. Physiol. 17:*9–13 (1962).

5. West, J. B., and Dollery, C. T., Distribution of blood flow and ventilation–perfusion ratio in the lung, measured with radioactive CO_2, *J. Appl. Physiol. 15:*405–410 (1960).

6. Dollery, C. T., Heimberg, P., and Hugh-Jones, P., The relationship between blood flow and clearance rate of radioactive carbon dioxide and oxygen in normal and oedematous lungs, *J. Physiol. 162:*93–104 (1962).

7. Kenny, P. J., Watson, D. D., Janowitz, W. R., *et al.*, Dosimetry of some accelerator produced radioactive gases, *Proceedings of Radiopharmaceutical Dosimetry Symposium,* Oak Ridge (April 1976).

8. Buckingham, P. D., and Forse, G. R., The preparation and processing of radioactive gases for clinical use, *Int. J. Appl. Radiat. Isot. 14:*439–445 (1963).

9. Watson, D. D., Kenny, P. J., Gelband, H., *et al.*, A noninvasive technique for the study of cardiac hemodynamics utilizing $C^{15}O_2$ inhalation, *Radiology* (1976).

10. Jones, T., Levene, D. L., and Green, R., Use of carbon dioxide for inhalation radiocardiograms and measurements of myocardial perfusion, in: *Dynamic Studies with Radioisotopes in Medicine,* pp. 751–764, IAEA, Vienna (1971).

11. Matthews, C. M. E., Dollery, C. T., Clark, J. C., *et al.*, Radioactive gases, in: *Radioactive Pharmaceuticals,* Oak Ridge Institute of Nuclear Studies, Oak Ridge (April 1966).

Radioactive Gases in the Evaluation of Left Ventricular Function

R. J. Nickles, P. J. Nelson, R. E. Polcyn,

J. E. Holden, and A. J. Kiuru

Introduction

The hydrodynamic performance of heart chambers can be noninvasively investigated by quantitative evaluation of tracer dilution curves. The application of nuclear medical procedures to cardiac dynamic measurements must begin with two fundamental decisions concerning the radiotracer and the detection system, chosen to measure the desired cardiac parameter with the greatest sensitivity. After these choices have been made, the statistical quality of the data will dictate the level of refinement that is justified in the quantitative modeling of the heart as a pump. In particular, the measurement of atrial and ventricular ejection fractions and detection of valvular insufficiencies stand apart from most nuclear medical procedures due to the severe demands placed on spatial and temporal resolution. Accurate diagnosis can hinge on seeing count-rate differences of several percent in successive 10 cm^2 × 10 msec image slices, suggesting that observed data rates from the heart alone should be of the order of 1 MHz. The fundamental tracer/detector choices determine how far short of this ideal a practical procedure will fall.

The Anger camera or autofluoroscope interfaced to a digital data processor with megaword mass-storage capabilities is well suited for cardiac dynamic imaging with ^{99m}Tc-labeled pharmaceuticals. Absorbed dose to the patient, cam-

R. J. NICKLES, P. J. NELSON, R. E. POLCYN, J. E. HOLDEN, and A. J. KIURU · Department of Radiology, University of Wisconsin Medical School, Madison, Wisconsin

era pulse pileup, and A/D conversion times conspire to limit clinically useful total-image count rates to less than 70 kHz. The peak fraction of this activity that is resident in a given heart chamber postinjection reflects the sophistication of the injection technique. The high temporal contrast resulting from an injection via a wedged pulmonary arterial catheter[1] results in peak left ventricular count rates of the order of 10 kHz.[2] This ventricular count rate drops in half with a less invasive, flushed IV injection of the equivalent activity, as shown in Figure 1. A more serious objection is the wide time dispersion of the bolus passing through the left heart chambers, introducing complications in the evaluation of cardiac parameters from dilution curves.

Probe arrays multiscaled in a digital data processor offer the option of slicing the spatial–temporal dependence of a tracer distribution in a radically different way. Ventricular photopeak count rates can be pushed above 300 kHz, meaning that statistically meaningful data can be accumulated on a millisecond time scale. This temporal detail is preserved with only modest core requirements, reflecting the fact that the region-of-interest selection was performed a priori through probe position and collimation. It is just this single-channel nature of spatial interrogation that mars the probe approach. No amount of careful pericardial transmission imaging with fiducial markers will convince the image-oriented clinician that the probe field of view accurately encompasses the desired heart chamber.

It is worthwhile to remember that an image is an intermediate in ejection-fraction evaluation, and its need is relaxed as the tracer input-bolus dispersion is reduced to a point in space and time. Imagine that a spike of activity miraculously appears in the left ventricular blood pool via a catheter or ^{13}N-activation from a negative pion beam burst. Ejection fractions and valvular patency could be reliably evaluated from probe data, since the dilution curve could be modeled without reference to antecedent temporal structure.

The lungs are the closest input upstream of the left heart that can be noninvasively utilized. The inhalation of a highly soluble tracer gas represents a spatially diffuse, temporally compact injection into the pulmonary capillary blood with bolus dispersion at the left ventricle, depending on the inspiratory maneuver. Carbon dioxide,[3] labeled with ^{15}O ($t_{1/2} = 2$ min, β^+), crosses the alveolar membrane in fractions of a second,[4] transferring its label to blood water via enzyme catalysis. In a very practical sense, the properties of $C^{15}O_2$ are matched to cardiac probes in the same way that ^{99m}Tc seems to have been designed for the Anger camera. First, the input bolus is crisp, and the exiting label does not return from the systemic circulation. Second, the high count-rate capabilities of probes can be exploited, since the short half-life ensures that the patient can safely tolerate large administered activities. Likewise, ^{15}O is forgiving of probe-positioning errors, since the test can be repeated in minutes. Finally, the β^+ annihilation quanta can be tightly collimated by coincidence detection.

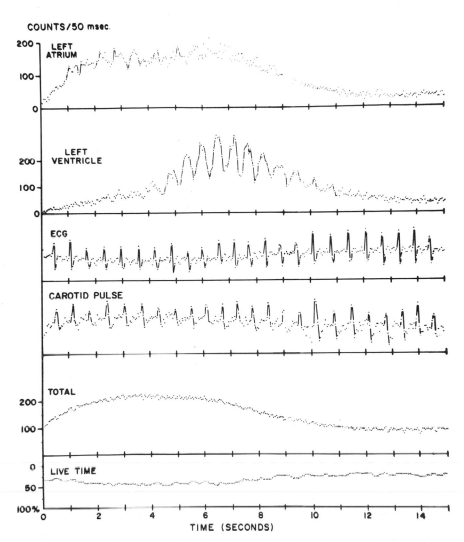

FIGURE 1 Cardiac dynamic study of a flushed IV injection of 10 mCi $^{99m}TcO_4^-$ collected at 20 images/sec in the LAO projection. From the top: LEFT ATRIAL count rate, contaminated with right heart activity; LEFT VENTRICULAR count rate; Parallel ECG; Parallel CAROTID PULSE; TOTAL observed count rate; system LIVE TIME, as measured by a constant-frequency pulser (see the text).

At the University of Wisconsin, the tracer/detector decision has been to develop both ^{15}O/probe and ^{99m}Tc/camera capabilities in an effort to investigate cardiac dynamics with high temporal and spatial detail, respectively.

Experimental Facilities

Radiotracer Production   A facility for the production of short-lived gaseous radiotracers has been developed in response to a growing interest in pulmonary-cardiovascular research.[4,5] The synthesis of ^{15}O-labeled gases warrants a brief description, since a similar approach could be employed by a number of nuclear medical groups not enjoying the luxury of an in-house cyclotron.

Production and Transport.   Carrier-free ^{15}O is produced through the ^{14}N (d, n) ^{15}O reaction utilizing a Tandem Van de Graaff accelerator in the UW Physics Department. The low-beam currents (several microamps on target) and the $\frac{1}{3}$-mile accelerator-clinic separation make optimal gas transport mandatory. A number of Teflon capillaries, ranging from $\frac{1}{2}$ mm to 3 mm ID, are "tuned" to transport maximal specific activities of various radionuclides to the receiving end in the nuclear medicine radiopharmacy, shown schematically in Figure 2. Bolus transmission suitable for the bulk of the heart studies results in the reception of 25 mCi ^{15}O/μA on target, while steady-state transmission can *maintain* about 10% of this activity in a 1-liter volume.

Radiochemistry.   The synthesis of $C^{15}O_2$ and $C^{15}O$ follows closely the work of the Hammersmith group.[6] A newly developed target chamber permits the on-line monitoring of target current, pressure, electron density, temperature, β^+ activity, and beam-induced optical spectra in an effort to gain understanding of the initial ion-molecular reactions that determine $^{15}O_2$ scavenging efficiency. Provisions have been made to perform in-target RF pumping of the intermediary excited O_2 molecular states that dominate the ^{15}O-trapping. Analysis of all radioactive gases make use of gas radiochromatography and differential trapping.

Gamma Detection Instrumentation

Imaging.   Dynamic image data are derived from either of two Anger cameras (Nuclear Chicago HP or Nuclear Data Radicamera II) interfaced with a PDP 11/40 computer with 28K of core and a pair of 1.2 megaword discs. Static, dynamic, or list-mode studies can be routinely performed with the foreknowledge that disk-write times alone place an upper limit of 70 kHz for loss-free data acquisition. In practice, an experiment requiring list-mode data rates greater than 50 kHz should be first mocked up by acquiring a scratch study of the entire injectate moving in the camera field of view.

Nonimaging.   Probe data are generated by an eight-detector array, shown in Figure 3, in which seven 2 in.$\times$2 in. NaI detectors are interrogated for 511 ± 50 keV events in coincidence with a similar event detected in a 5 in. $\times$ 4

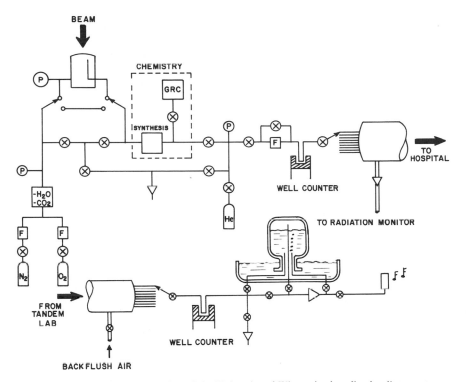

FIGURE 2. Schematic representation of the University of Wisconsin short-lived radiotracer transport system.

in. NaI detector. The time-to-amplitude convertor performs the dual function of ascertaining coincidence to within 8 nsec and analogue multiplexing of the coincident pair into computer core through blind scalers resident in a dedicated CAMAC crate. Singles and coincidence time–activity curves are multiscaled under software control, stored on disk, and displayed in real time on a GT 44 graphics display processor.

High time-dispersion radiocardiograms mostly employ the single 5 in. × 4 in. detector viewing the left ventricle in the LA or LAO projection through a 4 cm (dia.) × 10 cm (deep) straight-bore collimator. Minimum detector shielding is 10 cm of lead, with a total weight of 400 kg. The PM tube is operated at low voltages and a double-delay line amplifier with 250-nsec shaping-time constants results in a 511±50 keV pulse-pair resolving time of 800 nsec. Losses at high count rates are monitored by injecting a constant-frequency, noisy pulser ($E_{Eq} = 1500±50$ keV) into the preamplifier test input. System live-time is proportional to the pulser count rate passing through the 100 keV window.

Biotelemetry. Physiological data are needed in parallel with the radiocar-

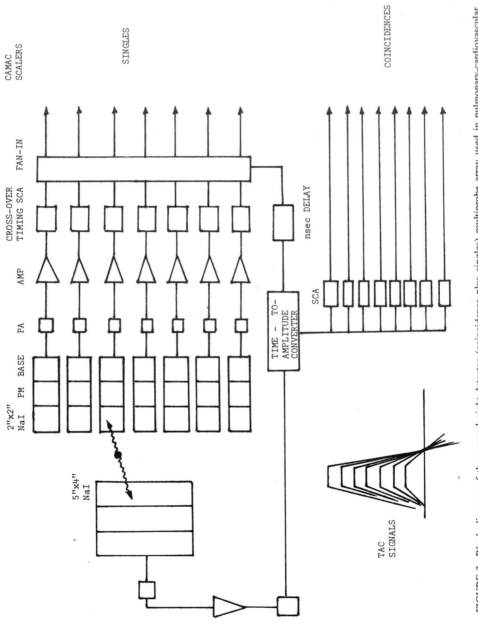

FIGURE 3. Block diagram of the general eight-detector (coincidence plus singles) multiprobe array used in pulmonary-cardiovascular studies with positron-emitting radionuclides.

diogram to provide an intrinsic cardiac clock for subsequent data analysis. Pneumotach, ECG, and carotid pressure states are recorded within individual frames of a dynamic study by frequency-modulating tail pulsers whose outputs mimic the photoevent of the tracer being imaged. These pulse trains are injected into test-pulse inputs installed in the preamps servicing the outer PM ring of the gamma camera head, as shown in Figures 4 and 5. The resulting physiological parameters appear as image points outside the camera field of view. Region-of-interest selection around these peaks generates time–activity curves in temporal synchrony with the radiotracer distribution. A constant frequency pulser, similarly injected, monitors system live-time. Biotelemetry with probes is simply a matter of multiscaling the appropriate voltage-frequency converters via the CAMAC scalers.

Results

Preliminary studies have been performed on 4 normal volunteers, and $C^{15}O_2/^{99m}Tc$ results will be shown for 1 subject (author, R. J. Nickles) to compare ejection/fraction analysis techniques. Figures 6 and 7 show the right lung apex and the left ventricular count rates following rapid inhalation of roughly 10

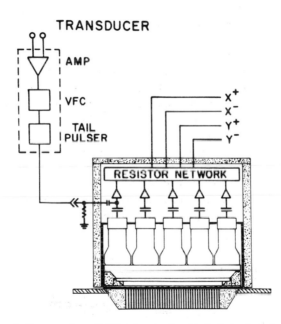

FIGURE 4. Schematic diagram of parallel biotelemetry input to include physiological (e.g., ECG) data into gamma-camera dynamic studies.

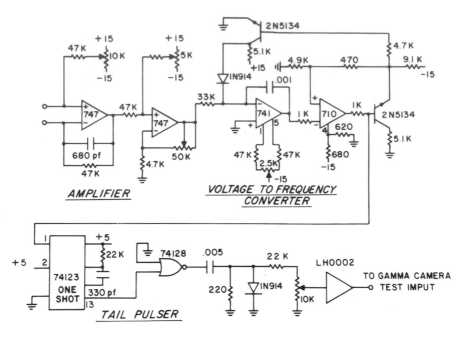

FIGURE 5. Diagram of generalized biotelemetry circuit. Voltage signals from a transducer frequency-modulate a tail pulser for input into the gamma-camera head.

mCi $C^{15}O_2$. The high time dispersion is necessary to observe the temporal detail in individual cardiac cycles. Likewise, the 250 kHz count rates are barely sufficient for high statistical precision at these sampling rates. Figure 8 demonstrates the inhalation radiocardiogram following inhalation of a similar dose of $C^{15}O$. Visual comparison of $^{99m}Tc/C^{15}O_2/C^{15}O$ data of Figures 1, 6, and 8 emphasize the $C^{15}O_2$ bolus simplicity, which is a direct result of the proximal injection and absence of recirculation. Approximate evaluation of ventricular ejection fraction $f_V = 0.6$ can be performed by inspection of Figure 7 over the "stair-step" systolic descent at the bolus trailing edge (7th to 10th observed cardiac cycles). All data shown are uncorrected for decay (negligible) or count-rate losses, which require a 50% correction for the ^{99m}Tc and 20% correction for the $C^{15}O_2$ data, respectively.

Analysis of Ejection Fractions

The upper "fitted" RCG of Figure 6 is the result of a nonlinear least-square analysis[7] seeking nine model parameters characterizing:
1. Pericardial background (3 parameters).
2. The distribution function K of Figure 9, representing the spread in lung-to-atrium delays (3 parameters).

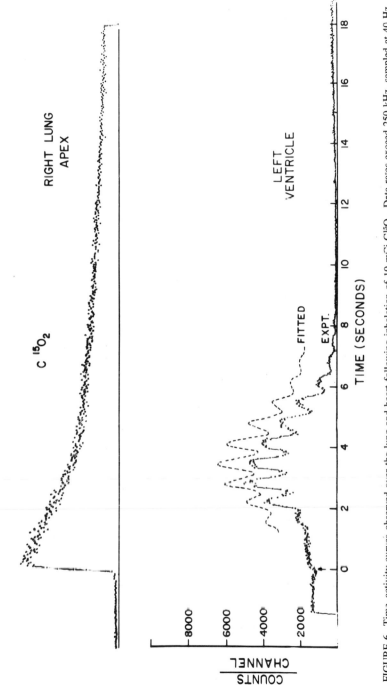

FIGURE 6. Time-activity curves observed over the lung and heart following inhalation of 10 mCi $C^{15}O_2$. Data rates exceed 250 kHz, sampled at 40 Hz. "Fitted" RCG represents model prediction with best-fit $f_A = 0.65(5)$, $f_V = 0.62(4)$.

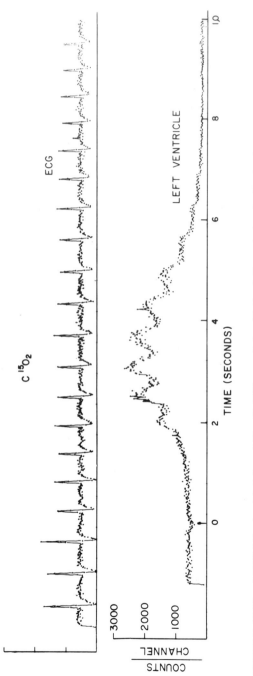

FIGURE 7. RCG and ECG following inhalation of 12 mCi $C^{15}O_2$ sampled at 80 Hz. Left-ventricular ejection fraction is approximately $f_V = 0.6$ from inspection at $5 \leqslant t \leqslant 7$ sec.

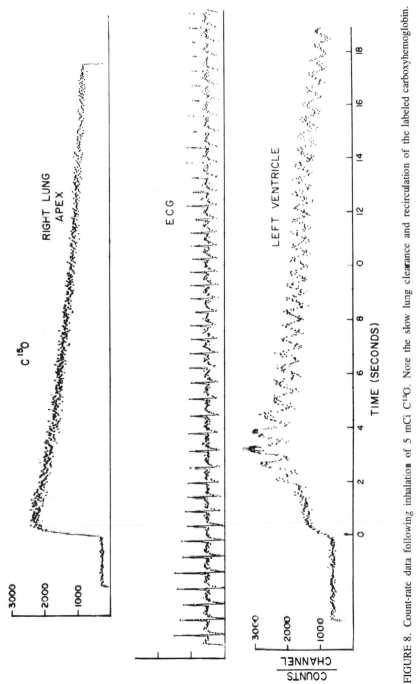

FIGURE 8. Count-rate data following inhalation of 5 mCi $C^{15}O$. Note the slow lung clearance and recirculation of the labeled carboxyhemoglobin. Cardiac output analysis hinges on comparison of first-pass to equilibrium activities.

3. Left atrial and ventricular ejection fractions f_A and f_V (2 parameters).
4. The extent to which the left atrium lies in the ventricular field of view (1 parameter).

The fit shown assumes a quadratic background and Gaussian kernel K acting as the Green's function in the integral convolution generating the bolus time dependence $B(t)$ upstream of the atrial input. The two ejection fractions enter through the four recursion relations of Table 1, coupling end-diastolic/systolic and atrial/ventricular activities. The search quickly converges to the best-fit values $f_A = 0.65$ (5), $f_V = 0.62$ (4) for the two measurements shown. Application of the Freedman[8] technique to the data of Figure 6 gives $f_V = 0.67$, showing the

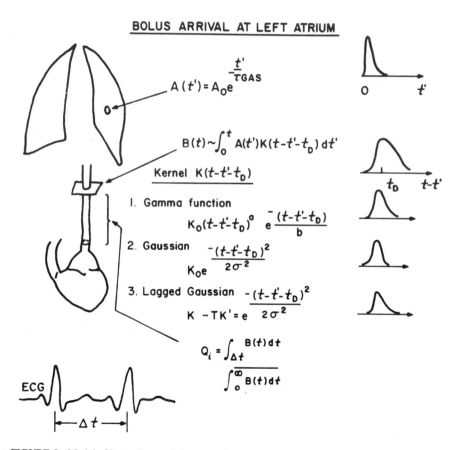

BOLUS ARRIVAL AT LEFT ATRIUM

$$A(t') = A_0 e^{-\frac{t'}{\tau GAS}}$$

$$B(t) \sim \int_0^t A(t')K(t-t'-t_D)\,dt'$$

Kernel $K(t-t'-t_D)$

1. Gamma function
$$K_0(t-t'-t_D)^a \; e^{-\frac{(t-t'-t_D)}{b}}$$

2. Gaussian
$$K_0 e^{-\frac{(t-t'-t_D)^2}{2\sigma^2}}$$

3. Lagged Gaussian
$$K - TK' = e^{-\frac{(t-t'-t_D)^2}{2\sigma^2}}$$

$$Q_i = \frac{\int_{\Delta t} B(t)\,dt}{\int_0^\infty B(t)\,dt}$$

ECG

$\leftarrow \Delta t \rightarrow$

FIGURE 9. Model of input charges Q_i incrementing the activity in cardiac blood pools. The kernel K represents the distribution in lung-atrium delays, smearing the fast injection of $C^{15}O_2$ across the alveolar membrane.

TABLE 1. Left Heart Chamber End-Point Activity Recursion Relations

Chamber	End-diastole[a]	End-systole[a]
Left atrium	$R_i = S_{i-1} + Q_i$	$S_i = R_i (1 - f_A)$
Left ventricle	$T_i = U_{i-1} + R_i f_A$	$U_i = T_i (1 - f_V)$

[a]In these equations, f_A is the left atrial forward-ejection fraction, f_V is the left ventricular forward-ejection fraction.

internal consistency between the two approaches. The ^{99m}Tc results of Figure 1 show $f_V = 0.51$ (4) simply from subtraction of carefully summed end-diastolic and end-systolic images. The Freedman approach yields a value of $f_V = 0.59$.

The model subroutine, describing the ventricular activity, is being upgraded in a number of details. Pericardial background will be measured and scaled to provide more credible baselines than an arbitrary analytic function. Lagged Gaussian[9] and gamma variates[10,11] are all being examined to describe the kernel K in the integral transform of Figure 9. Valvular insufficiencies will be allowed.[2] But, primarily, the suggestion of Ishii and MacIntyre[12] of fitting several vascular sections simultaneously is being incorporated into a global model that demands self-consistency in predicting tracer flow through serially related mixing chambers.

Conclusions

Our experience indicates that $C^{15}O_2$ inhalation radiocardiograms can play an important role in the evaluation of left ventricular function. Ideally, the $C^{15}O_2$/camera combination would allow cardiac imaging with high spatial *and* temporal detail. Data-rate limitations presently force us to employ the ^{99m}Tc/camera and $C^{15}O_2$/probe alternatives to separately achieve these goals. The two techniques are entirely complementary, illuminating cardiac flow patterns from different perspectives. The cardiac model that can successfully predict both tracer dilution curves warrants our most serious attention.

Acknowledgments

It is a pleasure to thank R. Morin and R. Wery for their assistance in this project, as well as the University of Wisconsin Nuclear Physics group for their generous allocation of beam time. Gratitude is also due the USAEC [Contract AT (11-1) GEN-7] and the James A. Picker Foundation.

References

1. Steele, P. P., Kirch, D. L., Mathews, M. E., and Davies, H., Measurement of left heart ejection fraction and end diastolic volume by a computerized scintigraphic technique using a wedged pulmonary artery catheter, *Amer. J. Cardiol. 34:*179 (1974).

2. Kirch, D. L., Metz, C. E., and Steele, P. P., Quantitation of valvular insufficiency by computerized radionuclide angiocardiography, *Amer. J. Cardiol. 34:*711 (1974).

3. Jones, T., Levene, D. L., and Greene, R., Use of ^{15}O-labeled carbon dioxide for inhalation radiocardiograms and measurements of myocardial perfusion, in: *Dynamic Studies with Radionuclides in Medicine,* IAEA, Vienna (1971).

4. West, J. B., and Dollery, C. T., Uptake of ^{15}O-labelled CO_2 compared with ^{11}C-labelled CO_2 in the Lung, *J. Appl. Physiol. 17:*9 (1962).

5. Nickles, R. J., and Au, Y. F., The oxygen clock—A dual tracer physiological Timer, *Phys. Med. Biol. 20:*54 (1975).

6. Glass, H. I., and Sylvester, D. J., Cyclotrons in nuclear medicine, *Brit. J. Radiol. 43:*589 (1970).

7. Bevington, P. R., Subroutine CURFIT, in: *Data Reduction and Error Analysis for the Physical Sciences,* p. 237, McGraw-Hill, New York (1969).

8. Freedman, G. S., Dwyer, A., Lange, R., Puri, S., Wolfson, S., Zaret, B., and Wolberg, J., Evaluation of ejection fraction using mathematical determination of background curve from the radiocardiogram, 60th Meeting of R. S. N. A., No. 123, Chicago (December 1974).

9. Bassingthwaite, J. P., Plasma indicator dispersion in the arteries of the human leg, *Circ. Res. 19:*332 (1966).

10. Thompson, H. K., Starmer, C. F., Whalen, R. E., and McIntosh, H. D., Indicator transit time considered as a gamma variate, *Circ. Res. 14:*502 (1964).

11. Kuikka, J., Lehtovirta, P., Kuikka, E., and Rekonen, A., Application of the modified gamma function to the circulation of cardiopulmonary blood pools in radiocardiography, *Phys. Med. Biol. 19:*692 (1974).

12. Ishii, Y., and MacIntyre, W. J., Analytical approach to dynamic radioisotope recording, *J. Nucl. Med. 12:*792 (1971).

Early Effect of Cardiac Surgery on Left-Ventricular Ejection Fraction

Peter Steele, George Pappas, Michael Jenkins,
Gerry Maddoux, and Dennis Kirch

Introduction

Aortocoronary artery bypass (ACB) is being performed with increased frequency for the relief of angina in patients with coronary artery disease.[1,2] Despite the satisfactory relief of angina, however, there has been concern that the operation may be associated with either deterioration or lack of improvement in left ventricular (LV) performance.[3-6] In addition, there is a definite risk of intraoperative acute myocardial infarction.[7-8] Also, low cardiac output is frequently observed early after valve replacement surgery, and this may reflect LV dysfunction. Considerable attention has been paid to optimal preservation of myocardium in patients undergoing cardiac surgical procedures.

Recently, we utilized intraaortic balloon pumping (IABP) during cardiopulmonary bypass to achieve pulsatile blood flow with the hope of providing a more physiologic myocardial blood-flow pattern during cardiopulmonary bypass with subsequent preservation of organ function.[9] This concept might be particularly useful when applied to the ischemic and thus threatened myocardium of patients with coronary artery disease (CAD), in that myocardium might be preserved if (PF) was present during cardiopulmonary bypass.

The purpose of this investigation was to measure left-ventricular ejection

PETER STEELE, GEORGE PAPPAS, MICHAEL JENKINS, GERRY MADDOUX, and DENNIS KIRCH · Department of Medicine and Department of Surgery, Denver Veterans Administration Hospital, University of Colorado Medical Center, Denver, Colorado.

fraction (LVEF) in patients undergoing cardiac surgery before and early after (1–12 days) the procedure. In patients undergoing ACB grafting, PF during cardiopulmonary bypass was compared to nonpulsatile flow. In addition, the outcome of patients receiving pulsatile myocardial flow during cardiopulmonary bypass was compared with that of patients not receiving PF.

Methods

Eighteen men undergoing aortic valve replacement with either directly sewn or stented aortic homografts were studied.[10] Fifteen men who had an open procedure on the mitral valve—commissurotomy in 6, mitral replacement in 9—were also studied. Of the commissurotomy patients, none had more than minor mitral regurgitation either pre- or postoperatively, and none of the mitral replacement or aortic-valve replacement patients had mitral or aortic regurgitation postoperatively. Mitral replacements included unstented aortic homografts[11] or stent-mounted porcine aortic valves.

Forty men undergoing ACB surgery were studied. These men constituted a consecutive series of patients operated on at the Denver Veterans Administration Hospital either for stable or preinfarction angina, but excluded patients requiring IABP prior to operation (patients with cardiogenic shock or pulmonary edema). In these 40 patients, 78 saphenous vein grafts and 4 internal mammary artery grafts were constructed.

IABP was performed, using an AVCO pump inserted via either a femoral artery or the ascending aorta, such that the balloon lay in the descending thoracic aorta. The left radial artery was cannulated to establish that diastolic augmention was occurring and to ensure that the left subclavian artery flow was not compromised by inadvertent balloon placement. The pump was sequenced with the ECG when sinus rhythm was present or to a cardiac pacemaker artifact when sinus rhythm was absent. IABP was begun at the time of cardiopulmonary bypass and discontinued following decannulation in all patients. In no case was postoperative IABP required, and none of these patients received sympathomimetic agents during the early postoperative period.

LVEF was measured preoperatively at the time of left cineventriculography and coronary cineangiography, again on the evening prior to surgery, and then serially following the operation beginning in the afternoon of the operation. Two studies were performed per day for the first 4 or 5 days, and a study was performed between 8 and 12 days postoperatively (day 10 study) (Tables 1 and 2). In the valve surgery, studies were also performed prior to surgery and over the first 10 days.

LVEF was measured by a radionuclide technique using ^{113m}In and a collimated scintillation probe.[12] The probe is portable, and all studies were done at the bedside. This method measures LVEF by recording a high-frequency

TABLE 1. Patients Operated on Without Intraaortic Balloon Pumping

Patient	Preop infarction	Preop LVEF[a] (%)		Postop LVEF[a] (%)		Postop infarction	Postop ischemic injury	Comment[b]
		LV cine	Radio	Day 1	Day 10±2			
1	+	46	56	60	60	0	0	Left main
2	+	—	66	50	50	0	0	Died, 3rd day
3	+	31	42	20	—	—	—	
4	+	42	37	20	25	0	0	
5	+	59	68	35	48	0	0	
6	+	51	58	40	35	0	0	
7	0	43	55	37	45	0	0	
8	+	20	20	20	20	0	0	
9	0	48	51	50	45	0	0	
10	0	56	60	68	68	0	+	Preinfarction
11	0	—	49	33	39	+	0	
12	+	61	55	45	55	0	0	
13	+	48	37	35	35	0	0	
14	0	79	60	41	63	0	+	Left main, preinfarction
15	+	20	25	20	20	0	0	
16	+	48	60	60	60	0	0	
17	+	—	44	50	53	0	0	
18	+	—	40	35	40	0	0	
19	0	—	43	25	30	0	0	
20	+	—	58	30	36	+	0	Left main, preinfarction
Mean ± SEM:		46.1±4.2	52.2±2.9	38.7±3.2 $P<0.001$	43.0±3.4 $P<0.001$			

[a] LVEF: Left-ventricular ejection fraction as measured from contrast ventriculogram (LV cine) and from radiocardiography (Radio).
[b] Left main indicates a left main coronary obstruction of >50%; Preinfarction indicates preinfarction angina.

TABLE 2 Patients Operated on With Intraaortic Balloon Pumping

Patient	Preop infarction	Preop LVEF[a] (%)		Postop LVEF[a] (%)		Postop infarction	Postop ischemic injury	Comment[b]
		LV cine	Radio	Day 1	Day 10±2			
1	0	—	44	57	60	0	0	
2	0	88	80	75	80	0	0	Left main
3	+	33	36	40	45	0	0	Left main
4	0	—	49	60	66	0	0	Left main
5	+	48	54	75	75	0	0	
6	+	41	53	59	60	0	0	Preinfarction
7	+	—	58	67	70	0	0	
8	+	—	41	46	49	0	0	
9	0	79	70	75	80	0	0	
10	+	53	56	57	63	+	0	
11	0	47	55	78	80	+	0	
12	+	39	40	53	58	0	0	
13	+	48	37	20	35	0	0	
14	+	28	25	48	50	0	+	Preinfarction
15	+	—	37	65	75	0	+	Left main, preinfarction
16	0	—	58	75	75	0	0	
17	0	60	66	70	75	0	0	
18	0	63	67	77	80	0	0	Prinzmetal
19	+	—	53	75	75	0	0	
20	+	—	49	60	65	0	0	
Mean ± SEM:		52.2±5.1	51.4±3.0	61.6±3.4 $P<0.001$	65.8±219 $P<0.001$			

[a]LVEF: Left-ventricular ejection fraction as measured from contrast ventriculogram (LV cine) and from radiocardiography (Radio).
[b]*Left main* indicates a left main coronary obstruction of >50%; *Preinfarction* indicates preinfarction angina; *Prinzmetal* indicate a patient with variant angina.

background-corrected time–activity curve from the left ventricle (Figure 1). Cardiac output was calculated from the radiocardiogram using radionuclide dilution concepts and the blood volume.[12] We have previously shown that LVEF measured with the scintillation probe correlates ($r = 0.90$ $N = 36$) with LVEF measured from the left cineventriculogram, and that cardiac output measured with [113mIn] and the probe correlates with cardiac output measured with indocynanine green dye ($r = 0.78$; $N = 35$).[12]

Of these 40 patients with CAD, 26 had a cineventriculogram adequate for determination of LVEF and LV end-diastolic volume (LVEDV) and a scintillation-probe study performed at the time of coronary angiography. Ventriculography was performed in the right anterior oblique projection by injecting 48 ml meglumine diatrizoate, 40% (renograffin, ER Squibb and Company), into the LV and filming at 60 frames/sec. Projected end-diastolic and end-systolic images were traced, and utilizing the planimetered area A and the LV long-axis (midpoint aorta to apex) L, the short axis M was calculated as[13,14]

$$M = \frac{2A}{\Pi} L$$

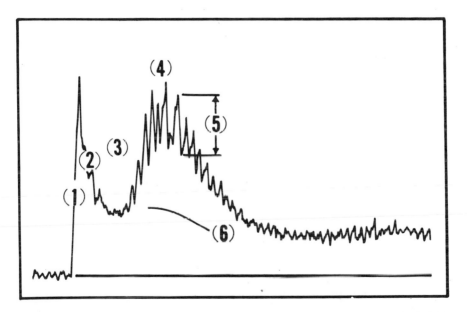

FIGURE 1. Precordial radiocardiogram to demonstrate the essential features of the bedside radionuclide technique: (1) Entry into right ventricle; (2) right ventricular washout; (3) radionuclide traversing the pulmonary circulation; (4) left ventricular peak; (5) fractional fall in count rate, end-diastole to end-systole; (6) mean of LV eclipse record (correction for radiation scatter) for calculation of LVEF. EF averages 50%; ratio end-diastolic to end-systolic count rate[5] to end-diastolic to eclipse line.[6]

and LVEDV calculated as

$$LVEDV = \frac{\Pi}{6} LM^2$$

The difference between LVEDV and LV end-systolic volume (stroke volume) divided by LVEDV yielded LVEF. A grid of 1-cm squares was filmed and used to correct for X-ray distortion.[15]

ECGs were recorded preoperatively and daily postoperatively. An acute myocardial infarction was diagnosed by ECG if a significant (0.04 sec), persistent (>10 days), new Q wave with typical ST and T wave changes were present. An ECG was categorized as ischemic injury if there was flat segment depression of > 2 mm or deep T inversion for 48 hr in the absence of a new Q wave.

Results

The 20 patients who had IABP during ACB surgery were comparable to the 20 who did not receive IABP in respect to preoperative radionuclide LVEF (mean ± SEM): 51.4±3.0% (Table 2) vs. 52.2±2.9% (Table 1). The two groups were also comparable with respect to history of preoperative myocardial infarction (60% vs. 70% of patients), and extent of CAD as assessed by the number of grafts received (38 vs. 44).

Preoperative LVEF (determined by radiocardiography) was depressed in both groups. In the 20 men who did not receive IABP, 10 (50%) had LVEF <55% (Table 1), and in the 20 who received IABP, 12 (60%) had LVEF <55% (Table 2). Correlation of radiocardiographic LVEF and cineventriculographic LVEF was good in the 26 patients who had both studies ($r = 0.86; P < 0.001$).

In the group that did not receive IABP, marked depression of LVEF was noted on the 1st postoperative day (52.2±2.9% to 38.7±3.2%), with some improvement noted by the 10th day (43.0±3.4%) (Table 1). But at day 10, there was still a significant ($P < 0.001$) decrement of LVEF vs. control (Figure 2). This early depression was not noted in the IABP group, and there was an increase in LVEF from 51.4±3.0% to 61.6±3.4% on day 1 ($P < 0.001$), and a further increase to 65.8±2.9% on day 10 (Table 2). In the non-IABP group, 8 of 20 (40%) had an increase of LVEF on day 1 as compared with the control, while in the IABP group, 17 of 20 (85%) had an increase on day 1.

The alteration of LVEF did show a relationship with preoperative myocardial infarction in the IABP group. An increase in LVEF occurred in 5 of the 12 (42%) with a history of myocardial infarction, but was increased in all 8 of the 8 without myocardial infarction. Alteration of LVEF was not related to the number of grafts placed. LVEF seemed quite strikingly altered in patients with preinfarctional angina who had IABP, but not in the preinfarctional patients who did not have IABP.

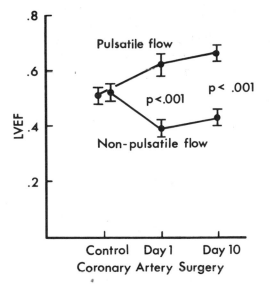

FIGURE 2. Favorable alteration in LVEF in patients undergoing coronary surgery with PF, as compared with patients with nonpulsatile flow during cardiopulmonary bypass.

Postoperative acute myocardial infarction occurred in 2 patients in each group (10%), and postoperative acute ischemic injury occurred in 2 in each group (10%). It is interesting to note that neither infarction nor ischemic injury was associated with depression of LVEF in either group. In fact, in the IABP group, 1 patient with infarction and 1 with ischemic injury had an actual increase of LVEF.

There was 1 death in the non-IABP group and no deaths in the IABP group. IABP was accomplished without complication in these patients.

Of the 18 men who underwent aortic valve replacement, LVEF was decreased on the 1st postoperative day in 13 (72%), and the average value fell significantly ($P < 0.001$) (from 52 ± 0.4 to $37 + 4\%$). Some reversibility of LVEF was noted: $39 \pm 4\%$ on day 2, $44 \pm 4\%$ on day 3. The value on the 3rd day remains significantly depressed compared with the preoperative value ($P < 0.001$). This early fall in LVEF did not correlate with preoperative LVEF, the presence of predominant or pure aortic stenosis, regurgitation, or mixed valve lesions. During aortic valve replacement, coronary perfusion was accomplished in all cases, but the aorta must, of necessity, be cross-clamped during valve insertion.

In the 15 men who underwent mitral surgery, average LVEF was reduced from a preoperative value of $52 \pm 4\%$ to $45 \pm 5\%$ on the 1st postoperative day ($P < 0.038$), and 10 of the 15 (67%) had some reduction in LVEF. Average values for LVEF did not increase on the 2nd ($45 \pm 5\%$) or 3rd ($46 \pm 5\%$) postoperative day. Of the 9 who underwent mitral replacement, 6 had a decrease in LVEF; of the 6 who had mitral commissurotomy, 4 had a decrease in LVEF. During mitral surgery, aortic cross-clamping, and consequent reduction in coronary blood flow, was required for variable periods of time to allow adequate visualization.

Thus, in patients undergoing valvular surgery in whom the circumstances require interruption of coronary flow, an early reduction in LV performance, as assessed by EF, frequently occurs. Some reversibility of LVEF seems to occur, particularly in patients following aortic valve replacement.

Discussion

The results suggest that LVEF in the early postoperative period is increased in patients undergoing coronary artery bypass surgery who have pulsatile myocardial blood flow during the surgical procedure.

The simple method of producing pulsatile myocardial and other organ perfusion using intraaortic balloon pumping seems to lessen myocardial injury during coronary artery surgery. Our data are in agreement with those of a number of other investigators who have shown that deterioration of LVEF occurs in association with coronary bypass surgery. In our patients who did not receive pulsatile myocardial flow, LVEF was decreased in the early postoperative period.

In this small series, pulsatile flow did not decrease the incidence of postoperative myocardial infarction or ischemic injury. It is of interest to note, however, that ECG evidence for infarction or injury was not necessarily associated with a decrement of LVEF. This probably reflects the occurrence of overall improvement in LV performance in association with a relatively small area of infarction. In a larger series, a decrease in the incidence of perioperative myocardial infarction might be apparent by pulsatile flow during coronary surgery.

In the pulsatile flow group, the data suggest than an increase in LVEF occurs primarily in patients without preoperative myocardial infarction, although LVEF can increase in patients with preoperative infarction. In the nonpulsatile group, no such relationship between preoperative myocardial infarction and change in LVEF was apparent.

The increase in LVEF in the pulsatile flow group probably results from improved myocardial blood flow or blood-flow distribution during cardiopulmonary bypass and thereby preservation of myocardium.[16,17] The improved preservation of myocardium during cardiopulmonary bypass would allow the reduced myocardial ischemia and consequently improve LV performance. This simple technique of producing pulsatile flow during cardiopulmonary bypass may be worth of consideration for coronary artery and other cardiac surgical procedures.

Acknowledgment

This work was supported by Veterans Administration Research Funds and a grant from the Colorado Heart Association.

The authors acknowledge the expert technical assistance of Mr. Michael LeFree, Wayne Whitney, Clyde Jordan, and Mrs. Gloria Smith and the secretarial assistance of Mrs. Peggy Corbin.

References

1. Favaloro, R. G., Saphenous vein graft in the surgical treatment of coronary artery disease: Operative technique, *J. Thorac. Cardiovasc. Surg. 58:*178 (1969).
2. Johnson, W. D., Flemma, R. J., Lepley, D., and Ellison, E. H., Extended treatment of severe coronary artery disease: A total surgical approach, *Ann. Surg. 170:*460 (1969).
3. Shepherd, R. L., Itscoitz, S. B., Glancy, D. L., Stinson, E. B., Reis, R. L., Olinger, R. N., Clark, C. E., and Epstein, S. E., Deterioration of myocardial function following aorto-coronary bypass operations, *Circulation 49:*467 (1974).
4. Arbogast, R., Solignac, A., and Bourassa, M. G., Influence of aortocoronary saphenous vein bypass surgery on left ventricular volumes and ejection fraction. Comparison before and one year after surgery in 51 patients, *Amer. J. Med. 54:*290 (1973).
5. Achuff, S., Griffith, L., Humphries, J. O., Conti, C. R., Browley, R., and Goff, V., Myocardial damage after aorto-coronary vein bypass surgery (abstract), *J. Clin. Invest. 51:*1a (1972).
6. Hammermeister, K. E., Kennedy, J. W., Hamilton, G. W., Stewart, D. K., Gould, K. L., Lipscomb, K., and Murry, J. A., Aortocoronary saphenous-vein bypass. Failure of successful grafting to improve resting left ventricular function in chronic angina, *N. Engl. J. Med. 290:*186 (1974).
7. Brewer, D. L., Bilbro, R. H., and Bartel, A. G., Myocardial infarction as a complication of coronary bypass surgery, *Circuation 47:*58 (1973).
8. Hultgren, H. N., Miyagawa, M., Buck, W., and Angell, W. V., Ischemic myocardial injury during coronary artery surgery, *Amer. Heart J. 82:*624 (1971).
9. Pappas, G., Winter, S. D., Kopriva, C. J., and Steele, P. P., Improvement of myocardial and other vital organ functions and metabolism with a simple method of pulsatile flow (IABP) during clinical cardiopulmonary bypass, *Surgery 77:*34 (1975).
10. Pappas, G., Blount, S. G., and Davies, H., Supported and non-supported valve homografts in man, *Ann. Thorac. Surg. 14:*513 (1972).
11. Yacoub, M. H., and Kittle, C. F., A new technique for replacement of the mitral valve by semilunar valve homograft, *J. Thorac. Cardiovasc. Surg. 58:*859 (1969).
12. Steele, P. P., Van Dyke, D., Trow, R. S., Anger, H. O., and Davies, H., Simple and safe bedside method for serial measurement of left ventricular ejection fraction, cardiac output and pulmonary blood volume, *Brt. Heart J. 36:*122 (1974).
13. Dodge, H. T., Sandler, H., Ballew, D. W., and Lord, J. D., The use of biplane angiocardiography for the measurement of left ventricular volume in man, *Amer. Heart J. 60:*762 (1960).
14. Kennedy, J. W., Trenholme, S. E., and Kasser, I. S., Left ventricular volume and mass from single plane cineangiocardiogram. A comparison of anteroposterior and right anterior oblique methods, *Amer. Heart J. 80:*343 (1970).
15. Greene, D. C., Carlisle, R., Grant, C., and Bunnell, I. L., Estimation of left ventricular volume by one plane cineangiography, *Circulation 35:*61 (1967).
16. Trinkle, J. K., Helton, N. E., Wood, R. E., and Bryant, L. R., Metabolic comparison of a new pulsatile pump and a roller pump for cardiopulmonary bypass, *J. Thorac. Cardiovasc. Surg. 58:*562 (1969).
17. Shepard, R. B., and Kirklin, J. W., Relation of pulsatile flow to oxygen consumption and other variables during cardio-pulmonary bypass, *J. Thorac. Cardiovasc. Surg. 58:*694 (1969).

Part V · Radioimmunoassay

Role of Radioimmunoassay in the Cardiac Patient—Principles and Applications

Fuad S. Ashkar

The English physician William Withering introduced digitalis therapy for the management of cardiac disorders around 200 years ago. Although the crude preparations were effective in heart failure, they were accompanied by gastrointestinal upset, visual disturbances, and often death. The dangers associated with digitalis therapy have continued to plague physicians until the present day, since they have had to contend with the narrow margin that exists between beneficial dosage and dosage resulting in toxicity, the variations in tolerance, absorption, excretion, sensitivity, and the lack of a sensitive assay for monitoring the drug blood and tissue levels.

The recent introduction of the radioimmunoassay (RIA) method for measuring blood levels of digitalis provided a useful, accurate guide for treatment that has resulted in a marked reduction in morbidity and mortality.[1] RIA uses antibodies of high affinity and specificity against specific cardiac glycosides.[2,3] In the presence of a fixed amount of radioactive-labeled digitalis, the digitalis in the patient's sample competes for reactive sites on the specific antiserum, after separation of the antibody-bound from the free digitalis. Levels in the patient's samples are determined by comparing the percentage of radioactivity bound to antibody with that in a series of standards. There is a fixed heart-to-blood digitalis ratio, at equilibrium 30:1, which allows monitoring tissue levels by measuring blood levels.

Following the oral administration of digitalis, there is a sharp rise in plasma

FUAD S. ASHKAR · Department of Radiology, University of Miami School of Medicine, Jackson Memorial Hospital, Miami, Florida.

levels within 15–30 min. A period of 4–6 hr is required for the level to fall to a plateau as the equilibrium between blood and tissue is established. Plasma digitalis concentration varies with the dose; the mean digoxin level in patients on long-term therapy is 1.4 ng/ml, ranging from 0.2 to 3.4 ng/ml, and toxic patients have a mean digoxin level of 3.3 ng/ml, with a range of 1.5–5.2 ng/ml. Although there is overlap in these levels, toxicity is always associated with levels over 2 ng/ml.[1-6]

TABLE 1. High-Risk Patients

Elderly	Associated pulmonary disease
Advanced heart disease	Abnormal thyroid status
Underlying atrial fibrillation	Acute myocardial infarction

TABLE 2. Factors That Cause Excess Digitalis Accumulation

Excessive dosage
Diminished excretion
  Renal disease
  Old age
  Hypothyroidism

TABLE 3. Factors That Increase Myocardial Sensitivity to Toxic Effects

Local factors
  Myocardial ischemia
  Myocardial disease
Systemic factors
    Hypokalemia
    Hypomagnesemia
    Hypercalcemia
  Anoxia
  Alkalosis
  Excessive circulating catecholamines
  Cardiopulmonary bypass

Findings from Clinical Studies

Of patients admitted to a medical service, 30% had evidence of toxic effects from digitalis, while 11% were underdigitalized.

Studies in experimental patients indicate that 60% of a lethal dose has been given when cardiac arrhythmias first appear.

Toxicity is common in high-risk patients (Table 1). Therapy in this group should be monitored closely and frequently.

Factors that cause excess digitalis accumulation (Table 2) should be investigated rapidly in patients showing toxic effects.

Numerous conditions, local and systemic, may increase myocardial sensitivity to digitalis (Table 3). Dose adjustment and correction of these factors should be made when feasible, and digitalis blood levels should be interpreted accordingly.

The frequent use of serum digitalis assay in clinical practice can decrease the frequency of adverse reactions to digitalis.[1-6]

References

1. Ashkar, F. S., *Practical Nuclear Medicine,* Medcom Press, New York (1974).
2. Butler, V. P. Jr., Digoxin: Immunologic approaches to measurement and reversal of toxicity, *N. Engl. J. Med. 383:*1150 (1970).
3. Doherty, J. E., The clinical pharmacology of digitalis glycosides: A review, *Amer. J. Med. Sci. 255:*382 (1968).
4. Duhme, D. W., Greenblatt, D. J., and Koch-Weser, J., Reduction of digoxin toxicity associated with measurement of serum levels, *Ann. Intern. Med. 80:*516 (1974).
5. Smith, T. W., Butler, V. P. Jr., and Harber, E., Determination of therapeutic and toxic serum digoxin concentration by radioimmunoassay, *N. Engl. J. Med. 281:*1212 (1969).
6. Smith, T. W., and Haver, E., Clinical value of serum digitalis glycoside concentrations in the evaluation of drug toxicity, *Ann. N. Y. Acad. Sci. 179:*322 (1971).

Index